JUNGLE
MEDICINE

JUNGLE MEDICINE

CONNIE GRAUDS

THE CENTER FOR
SPIRITED MEDICINE

It is an unfortunate reflection of our society that we are forced to publish disclaimers. In my opinion, this can only serve to separate us even more from spirit, from our lives, and from the medicine at our feet ...Connie Grauds

Jungle Medicine is meant to be a discussion of the importance of spirit in our health. It is not a substitute for professional medical care. We urge you to seek also the best medical resources to help you make informed decisions about the nature of your condition and your treatment options.

JUNGLE MEDICINE
Copyright © 2004 by Connie Grauds

Grauds, Connie.
    Jungle medicine / Connie Grauds. -- 2nd ed.
    p. cm.
    Includes bibliographical references.
    LCCN 2003115491
    ISBN 0-9747303-0-0

    1. Grauds, Connie. 2. Pharmacists--United States--
Biography. 3. Shamanism--Amazon River Valley.
I. Title.

RS73.G66A3 2004   615'.1'092
                           QBI03-200958

Book designed by Michael Saint James

Sacred Tree cover art from photographs
by Dennis McKenna, Michael Saint James and Connie Grauds

Published by
The Center for Spirited Medicine
P.O. Box 150727
San Rafael, CA 94915
(415) 479-1512

To my Mother ... bless you

To my Father ... thank you

In Memory

ACKNOWLEDGMENTS

This book has grown forth from the many petri dishes and fertile gardens of my life. I wish to thank my parents for inoculating me with the drive to work hard and persevere, invaluable qualities for the long and arduous task of book writing. I remember all of my family and the life we shared together in the resort town of Forest Lake, the Garden of Eden of my childhood. The love of those Minnesota forests and lakes of my youth has become the passion I have for the jungles and the rivers of the Amazon, my second home. My heartfelt thanks to my spiritual family—the people, the plants, and the spirits of the Amazon rainforest. It is my privilege to introduce you to some of them here in this book.

I am beholden to the College of Pharmacy at the University of Minnesota; for it is there that I became a true scientist—one who investigates the unknown through experimentation. I give thanks to two special colleagues, Dr. James Duke and Dr. Mark Plotkin, whose passion for the medicinal plants of the Amazon rainforest infected me, too; and also thanks to them both for introducing me to shaman don Antonio Montero Pisco.

Muchisimas gracias to don Antonio for being my healer, my friend, my *maestro*. His kindness, love, and gentleness of spirit showed me how to love life. His patience as a teacher allowed me to bloom gracefully. His toughness as a taskmaster showed me how to master my fears. From the bottom of my heart, I want to express my deepest gratitude to this truly remarkable man and gifted shaman. May I serve the medicine he has taught me with his same integrity.

I want to express a debt of gratitude to the other shamans and shamanas who have gone before me; special thanks to my friends and healers Elizabeth Jenkins, Thomas Pinkson and Eliot Cowan for lighting the path.

Thanks to the many other healers who have personally helped me along my path. I am especially indebted to Dr. Stanislav Grof and Dr. Ralph Metzner, whose pioneer work in altered states and transpersonal psychology showed me the transformative qualities of my spiritual experiences. I continue to pour heart-felt thanks and more thanks to Dr. Larry Dossey for his kindness of spirit and largess of support. Without his generous encouragement, I would not be where I am today.

A note of gratitude must go to all those who helped make this book a reality. I'm deeply beholden to my dear editor, Doug Childers, whose gifted talents transformed all of my scribblings and ramblings into a spirited story.

A special thanks to friend and colleague Dr. Dennis McKenna for the use of photographs from his own extensive work in the Amazon to contribute to the book art. I owe much to Martin Myman, Leona George-Davidson, and Jennifer McKeever whose special efforts kept my business and my life on course during this creative process. I want to acknowledge Mary Kundert, Kerry Hughes, and Kathie Klumpp for their willingness to review early manuscripts and help with the Spanish vocabulary, *gracias*.

I send my deepest gratitude wrapped in lots of love to Dean Grauds, my good friend and former husband. He has lived much of this story with me, and I thank him for being part of my life. Also many thanks to him, too, for his helpful literary guidance.

I would also like to acknowledge all of my friends, students, and colleagues for their support; special thanks to Dr. Lois Johnson, Susan Pomeroy, Christiane Diehnel, Carolyn Wolfe, Terry and Curtis. They remind me that no one can do life alone.

CONTENTS

INTRODUCTION

I'm a pharmacist who has worked in the world of conventional Western medicine for nearly thirty years, and I'm also a shamana who has apprenticed in the world of "non-rational" healing for nearly a decade. I stand with my feet firmly planted in two very different worlds.

This book tells the story of how my gradual disillusionment with my chosen profession, and a series of life-upheavals, including an extreme medical crisis—cancer—unexpectedly plunged me into profound and disturbing states of consciousness, encounters with the spirit world, and to my involvement in the healing arts of shamanism. During my apprenticeship to a powerful Amazon rainforest shaman, and in the course of my own peculiar ordeal, I learned deeper spiritual truths of healing which my previous medical training failed to provide. I also realized that the wealth of vital healing wisdom which the shamanic tradition offers could be combined with the technological wizardry of modern Western medicine to create a new paradigm of healing and health that encompasses the physical, mental, and spiritual domains.

Let me begin with a bit of personal background. I was born into a good Minnesota Catholic family in 1947, a time of renewed hope and prosperity. "The war to end all wars" had been won. My family owned a dry cleaners and lived beside one of the famed 10,000 lakes. Life for most people looked pretty good, at least on the outside. But people are also like lakes, their surfaces rarely show what is hidden in their depths.

When I was three years old, my family was plunged into dramatic and painful turmoil. The cause was my mother, whose hidden depths suddenly erupted to the surface in the form of literal insanity—so the doctors said. She began hearing unusual voices and seeing otherworldly visions. It was a confusing period for all of us. I mainly recall her strange behavior, and the fear that I felt when she was frightened. And I remember how, when her inner life overwhelmed her, she would retreat to the basement and hide in terror behind the furnace.

When I grew older, family members told me other details of her unusual behavior. Mother believed that she saw and spoke with otherworldly beings, and she'd talk giddily with monkey apparitions, and softly when angels were around. She was apparently psychic at times, and would announce who was at the front door before the doorbell rang. That she was usually right somehow made her seem all the more crazy and threatening to those around her.

The doctors said her condition was hormonal and would pass. It didn't. Drugs were prescribed, but failed to cure her. Eventually she was diagnosed as psychotic, put in a mental hospital, and given seventeen shock treatments for what ailed her. But the cure, as they say, was worse than the disease. The image of my shattered mother living out her life as an un-healed fragment of her former self, haunted me for years, as I'm sure it did everyone else who knew her.

It was my first unwitting glimpse of the tragic inadequacies of Western medicine.

There was great shame in our family about my "crazy" mother. We all tried our best to cover up both her craziness and our shame. As the oldest child, I felt my job was to look and act normal to the outside world—no doubt, on some deep level, for my own protection. I saw what they'd done to my mother for *not* being normal. I was taught early on that extraordinary voices and visions were signs of pathology, and that they would do bad things to you if you *ever* had them. And I did everything within my power to make sure that my life was grounded, rational, and above all, sane.

Not surprisingly, the sciences with their reassuring promise of certitude and control, became my passion. I grew to love the exactness and rigors of chemistry, biology and mathematics. In the eighth grade, I chose the profession of pharmacy as my life's calling. I imagine my choice was partly motivated by a hope that the life of a rational scientist would magically protect me from my mother's fate.

After graduating from the University of Minnesota's College of Pharmacy in 1969, my life was set. I became a pharmacist, a respected member of the Western medical establishment. Ironically, I had fled the fear of my mother's madness and its tragic consequences, into the arms of the healing profession that had virtually destroyed her because it could not comprehend the spiritual roots of her disease. In time, I would realize the medical profession was itself in need of spiritual healing.

We pharmacists love, and live in, the world of the exact.

The tablets in every bottle are numbered. Each of the many medications we dispense daily have a prescribed potency and a calculated effect. We fill prescriptions written by licensed physicians whose diagnoses are based on long-established medical procedures, consensus, and laboratory test results. The only "spirits" we encounter are distilled ones, measured in milliliters and bottled for sale. And we *never* talk to them.

But over the years I discovered innumerable cracks in this professional façade of exactitude, and I grew slowly disillusioned with pharmaceuticals and their "silver bullet" hype. I began to see how the medical world's dogmatic reliance on technology alone rests upon a consensus akin to faith, a worldview of limiting, inadequate assumptions about "the way things are."

Unacknowledged and unwelcome mysteries defy the apparent exactness, and haunt the rigid certitudes of modern medicine. For instance, why do some people die of apparently minor ailments, while others return from the brink of death or are inexplicably healed of chronic or terminal diseases? Where does the power of the healing process lie? Is it in the pills, powders, and elixirs? In the body that responds to them? In the mind of the patient? In the accumulated body of modern medical knowledge? Or does it perhaps lie elsewhere, in some unquantifiable realm of the soul where conventional medicine refuses to look, and which it disregards to its own impoverishment? All our medical theories and statistics, and our hopeful certainties, stand mute before these unanswered questions.

In my early forties, nearly two decades into my career,

my life began to fall apart. Disillusioned with my profession, my scientific certitude crumbling and my marriage of twenty years disintegrating, I learned that I had cancer of the thyroid and fell into a profound despair, a spiritual crisis that no conventional therapy and no prescription in my pharmaceutical bag of miracle drugs could cure. The scientific materialist worldview in which I had placed my faith, and on which I had founded my life, was no longer a support.

Through a series of seemingly random events, I ended up in the Amazon jungle. There I met a powerful rainforest shaman. What followed was an unexpected, disorienting plunge into the world of the irrational—a realm of inner visions and voices, powerful energies, and strange experiences.

At that point I knew nothing about shamanism, nor did I imagine my ordeal to be anything like an initiation. I experienced only the terror of madness, buried deep within me since childhood. And that child, still within me, seemed to say, "If I tell you who I really am and what I really think and see and hear and feel, you'll drug me and hurt me, you'll lock me up and tie me down and fry my brain with electricity…like you did to my mother." But my dark night of the soul proved to be the medicine I needed. And don Antonio, the shaman whose apprentice I became, proved to be the healer I needed.

Amazon jungle shamans are masters of the potent pharmacological healing properties of medicinal rainforest plants. They are also adept voyagers of the spirit world, the inner sea of the psyche. And they routinely help others to navigate this sea where countless accidental or unprepared Western voyagers like my mother, and me almost, have been shipwrecked and lost.

Shamans, by their experiential training and their spiritual worldview, are at home in non-ordinary realities that Western medicine typically pathologizes, often to the detriment of the patient. Shaman don Antonio understood what was happening to me and helped me to see it as a transformational, rather than a pathological, process. It made all the difference. He walked with me to the edges of madness where I wrestled with my inner demons. He helped me to understand and relate directly to those powers from which indigenous shamans, for centuries, have drawn their healing wisdom and spiritual gifts. In doing so, he initiated me into ancient mysteries of healing upon which modern medicine has turned its back.

I write this book out of such unusual experiences and perspectives—as a long-time pharmacist dispensing chemical medicines to suffering patients; as a former patient afflicted by potentially devastating physical and psychological conditions; and as a practicing shamana, a healer using a unique combination of "rational" and "irrational" medicine by which my own cancer was healed. My experiences have shown me that true healing is a multi-dimensional event, a mysterious transaction between the souls of doctor and patient, between medicine and the physical body, and between the patient and mysterious spirit realms which mystics and shamans have explored for ages.

For now, conventional Western medicine operates exclusively in the realms of intellect and matter, science and technology. The emotional/spiritual dimensions of our illnesses are rarely considered or attended to. This results in what I call "spiritless medicine." The frequency of misdiagnoses, malpractice, needless surgeries and prescriptions, illnesses contracted in hospitals, and indifferent healthcare environments, seem to be inevitable consequences of spiritless medicine. Not to mention countless frustrated, suffering people who are often not helped, and at times even harmed by their healthcare, and who sense that their profound spiritual needs have been exiled from the healing equation.

We in the medical profession habitually focus on symptoms. And our myopic focus on symptoms hides a peculiar blindness to the often emotional and spiritual origins of much illness. By treating symptoms as if they *were* the disease while ignoring significant "non-rational" factors, we unwittingly separate ourselves and our patients from a true healing process. We settle instead for damage control, for chemical bombardment of chronic ailments like high blood pressure, depression, hypertension, asthma, allergies, and many others. And the dogmatic adherence to this shortsighted approach reveals an emptiness at the core of modern medicine.

But it's gradually becoming clear to many of us, both in and out of the healing professions, that health is not a mere absence of symptoms, and that chemical warfare against symptoms cannot properly be called "healing." Part of us knows the power that heals is not in the elixirs, surgeries, and pills. We're all looking for the real *Medicine*, for true healing, for authentic, radiant health. But most of us, including our doctors, don't quite know how to find them.

And we can't blame everything on "the system," even if it is flawed. Can we blame our doctors for failing to cure us when we might have taken better care of ourselves? After-the-fact medical intervention is hardly a substitute for preventative measures such as a healthy diet, exercise, rest, and minimal bad habits.

Not all ailments are self-induced through irresponsible living. And given modern medicine's PR image of near-infallible authority, it's natural for people to be painfully disillusioned when they discover—while they are suffering, sick, or dying—that there is no certain diagnosis for what ails them, no magic pill to cure them, and that modern medical science is, after all, as fallible as the humans who practice it.

Part of me still believes wholeheartedly in the wonders of modern medicine. It has given new life to many through blood transfusions and organ transplants; abolished scourges like polio, smallpox, and tuberculosis; cured pneumonia, malaria, and other life-threatening illnesses with powerful antibiotics; repaired terrible injuries through surgical techniques; and done untold good to countless millions of people. But perhaps these truly staggering achievements have also led us into a kind of scientific/ materialistic hubris.

After three decades in the trenches of conventional Western medicine, my nagging sense is that it may be no more reliable, in terms of ultimate healing, than the methods of the indigenous shamans and spirit healers whom we love to discredit and deride, and from whom we could learn much, if we only would.

In this book I explore a new paradigm that integrates the best of these two honorable and legitimate healing traditions. I affirm the value of Western medicine, and also suggest how both patients and healers can look beyond pills and surgery for deeper answers to the dilemmas that every illness represents.

My vision and my experience tell me that these two seemingly incompatible healing traditions—one ancient and one modern—can meet and form a union more whole and powerful than their separate parts. My hope is that the information in this book, which saved and transformed my own life, may do the same for yours.

My prayer is that the unique wisdom of indigenous shamanism can help to heal a spiritual wound in the soul of modern Western medicine whose body—our health care system—is presently in crisis.

May we all help to create a new paradigm of spirited medicine practiced by spirited healers.

CHAPTER 1

TH€ JUNGL€
<ALL$

n 1994, on a day like any other in the life of an HMO clinic pharmacist, I scrambled to fill a thousand prescriptions for a room full of sick people. Weary by 10 A.M., I lifted my eyes from the dispensing counter to gaze at the long line of people waiting to hand me their prescriptions, and at the several dozen chairs where others sat waiting for their prescription 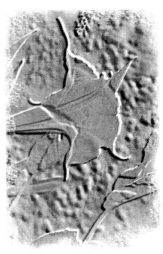 numbers to appear on the digital screen overhead. There were subdued, feverish looking kids, senior citizens, some supported by canes or walkers, a few looking isolated or depressed. Babies cried or squirmed in the arms of their stressed-out moms. Here and there I saw the random bandaged eye, or neck brace, or an arm or leg in a cast.

You couldn't tell, just by looking, why most of them had come. Their ailments were internal, and for many, chronic—an allergy, virus, or degenerative disease; a weak or malfunctioning organ; cancer; or perhaps the problem was even "in their heads." They came like dismal pilgrims to this modern healing grotto, seeking a magic pill or potion which they hoped would cure them. Yet too often their palliative prescriptions lacked the dose of hope which they needed most. More than a few of their faces and names were familiar to me. I'd been filling their prescriptions for years.

I'd started my career thinking my little Rx's could save the world one patient at a time. But I was soon cured of that comforting illusion. To those afflicted with chronic ailments, modern medicine can seem like a crapshoot, a sentiment voiced to me countless times over the years, often with a cynical despair rooted in painful personal experience. Today, for some reason, I was getting an earful of frustrated complaints. It started when Mrs. Anderson stepped up to the counter. I'd been refilling her blood pressure medication for over two years now.

"A refill today, Mrs. Anderson?" I'd asked.

"No, Connie," she'd answered. "I have two new prescriptions. My old blood pressure medication stopped working." She wrote her address on the new prescriptions for me and said, "I don't know about all this new medication. Doesn't my doctor know my blood pressure problem is in my head, not in my heart?" She sighed. "This medicine isn't going to fix what's going on in my head."

Tell that to your doctor and you'll get a third prescription for Prozac, I thought, indulging in a little cynical despair myself.

A few minutes later, Mr. DuPont, a stressed-out fifty-something exec in a local high-tech telecom company, stepped up to the counter. He fumbled for his membership healthcard with a pained, dispirited look. "I need a refill of this new headache medication," he said dully, then added, "All these medications seem to work for a while. Then they don't, and the headaches come right back. Why is it they can put some stranger's organ in you and make it work, but they can't cure a simple headache? I feel like I'm hitting my head against a wall."

Half an hour later, Mrs. Cusack, one of my favorites, stepped briskly up to the counter for a refill of her allergy medication. She plopped the empty bottle down onto the counter. She'd been coming here for over five years since her allergy tests had revealed that, as she put it, "I'm allergic to everything including oxygen. I should live in a plastic bubble and breathe allergy medication." Yet also according to her, her medication's side effects were only slightly less irritating than the allergies themselves.

"This stuff is practically worthless," she now said bluntly with her usual spunk. "But you can refill it anyhow. If you ask me, I'm really allergic to my husband."

That got a laugh out of her and me both. Who knew? It might be true!

Finally, a few minutes later, a glum Ms. Holland had come in for her bi-monthly refill. She suffered from a chronic depression, that the pills she took did not hide. Her prescriptions were chemical 'restraining orders' against inner demons that were clearly still tormenting her. She'd been started on Prozac two years ago, switched to Zoloft after six months, and switched to Paxil six months after that. There seemed to be as much guesswork as science involved in the matter. Today she'd seemed especially listless as she handed me another "new" prescription…Prozac again, the best of what didn't seem to be working very well. I knew she'd hoped the new miracle antidepressants would jump-start her back into life. I'd hoped the same. But she was trapped in a pharmaceutical foxhole on some inner battlefield.

So was I, in a different way—trapped in a room full of ailing, pain-wracked people whom I seemed unable to truly help. They waited for their prescription numbers to flash across a bingo board, then came through the chute where I spoonfed them pharmaceuticals like secular communion wafers. I had a brief, unpleasant image of myself as Nurse Ratched in "One Flew Over The Cuckoo's Nest," manually sticking pills under their tongues to keep them "manageable."

To what good end, I wondered? The pharmaceuticals I once thought could cure anything, I now regarded as chemical stun guns used, for the most part, to temporarily repress symptoms. For many, the symptoms reappeared when the pills ran out, and they returned to buy more. Repeat customers are the backbone of the business of modern medicine. My chosen career was beginning to look to me like mass pharmaceutical management, not healing.

I wondered how many patients felt, as Mrs. Anderson, that the system into whose hands they had put their health was systematically failing to address the root causes of their medical conditions. Many doctors seemed to view symptoms as autonomous facts, and their patients as biochemical machines. They made medical diagnoses, prescribed remedies, and even performed surgeries without deeply inquiring into their patient's lives to seek the complex core of the problem. Very much in the same way that I handed out pills.

A nagging sense was growing in me that there must be more to the healing process than routine office encounters and remedial chemical or surgical interventions. Every unhappy or worried or despairing patient's face told me that some vital human, perhaps even spiritual, component was also required for true healing to occur. And whatever it was could not be distilled in a laboratory or dispensed in a plastic bottle. And all the pills prescribed in its stead could not make up for its absence. Yet what *was* the elusive component? And how could it be provided by harried healthcare practitioners emotionally armored against the fear, pain, and vulnerability of their patients? How could it be provided by doctors who were often as bewildered, as much in need or in pain as their patients? Was there such a thing as "soul" and "spirit," and how did they fit into the healing equation?

These were the kinds of questions I'd recently begun asking myself. If I asked many of the doctors I knew such questions, it would raise their skeptical, scientific eyebrows, as it would have raised mine not too long ago, perhaps evoking a cynical response like, "It's not my department." Yet the last time I checked, there was no Soul Wing at the HMO clinic.

I remember how my faith in the myth of the "magic potion" had led me to choose a career in pharmacy in the eighth grade. My fascination with chemistry, mathematics, and biology had merged with my deep desire to help people who were suffering. I had felt called to the profession of pharmacy as some are called to the ministry. Instilled with a Protestant work ethic and an ingrained altruistic streak, I had imagined myself a 'Florence Nightingale' behind a prescription counter, healing minds and bodies, and saving lives by dispensing state-of-the-art medications. Science, that infallible authority, told me my vision was true. Yet it had also shown me, in my mother's case, that it was not.

My mother's ordeal had instilled in me a sensitivity to the suffering of others. And her madness, effectively suppressed through chemical means, had instilled in me a profound respect for the power of pharmaceuticals. Hadn't those "magic pills" brought her back from the depths of psychosis, an illness perhaps as mysterious and terrible as death itself? I was too young then to distinguish between "containment" and "cure." Only in the last few years had this distinction become painfully clear.

Behind me the robotics of pharmacy functioned with orderly precision in response to prescriptions. Counted pills and measured liquids tumbled into bottles, were put in paper bags, delivered to the front counter and handed to patients. In over twenty-four years as a practicing pharmacist I'd filled hundreds of thousands of prescriptions, dispensing a river of pills, ointments, and elixirs to a patient population the size of a modern metropolitan city. Each year I saw the waiting rooms getting fuller, and more medicines more than often not working. Meanwhile the vision of healing I had been called to serve was evaporating before my eyes.

Somehow listening to my patients' complaints today brought it all to a head.

I felt tired and disillusioned, like a weary foot soldier in the army of mechanized medicine. I knew I was fighting on the right side of the war. But I'd lost my faith in the generals.

I was almost ready for Prozac myself by the time my lunchbreak came. I grabbed my lunch bag from the fridge and headed for the exit. I needed to get outdoors, away from the pharmacy smells of alcohol, sulfur, medicines, vitamins, and cod-liver oil. On my way out, I glanced in my PO box near the time clock. A current pharmacy journal was waiting for me, and I took it with me to browse through while eating my lunch.

These days I tended to merely scan the new pharmacy journals, which I had once read almost religiously from cover to cover. But today, while thumbing through this issue, an unusual image caught my attention: an exotic, full-page, beautiful color photo of the Amazon rainforest. In the picture, an American ethnobotanist leaned over plant samples holding a note pad. Beside him stood a native shaman in a loincloth, high cheekbones riding his timeless face. It was a compelling image, and an intriguing juxtaposition...modern science and ancient wisdom. It was a lead photo for an article on ethnobotanical approaches to pharmaceutical drug discovery.

Captured by the picture and intrigued by the topic, I read this unusual article between bites of sandwich and gulps of soda. The article mentioned how the rainforests are among the last places on Earth where indigenous cultures still live relatively undisturbed in nature; where traditional jungle shamans still utilize their cultures' accumulated knowledge of the medicinal uses of jungle plants; and where this native healing tradition dated back long before the advent of modern medicine.

I had always regarded such native healing traditions as backward and superstitious, primitive at best in their efficacy. This attitude permeated the medical profession as I knew it. Now, as I read the article, I learned some surprising facts. For instance, 120 clinically useful prescription drugs worldwide are derived from plants, around 39% of which are used in the U.S.. And 47 of these 120 drugs are derived from plants native to the tropical rainforests. The rainforests, it seemed, were an important source of medicinal plants used to create modern pharmaceuticals. And these were just some of the plants used for centuries by native shaman healers.

My belief was that high-tech synthetic pharmaceuticals were inherently superior to natural medicines. But the article informed me that only 4% of the 47 drugs originating in the rainforest were currently produced through synthesis. It appeared that Mother Nature was a formidable chemist in her own right. Yet this "news to me" was apparently ancient healing wisdom to many native cultures.

This rainforest shaman in the photo represented a vital link between pharmacologically active plants, and their original medicinal uses. One of his ancestors, who knew how many centuries ago, had first discovered the healing power of various plants, and then put this knowledge to use. Perhaps these "simple uneducated" medicine men were sophisticated in ways we did not understand. This picture and this article belied the B-movie witch doctors of my childhood...images of half-mad, wild-eyed men in grass skirts with bones thrust through their noses, dancing around poisonous concoctions fuming over jungle fires.

Everything about the article—the lush, tropical beauty of the picture, the concept of natural pharmaceuticals, and an ancient and exotic healing tradition—jumped out at me. Unlike the glossy Madison-Avenue pharmaceutical ads, and dry scientific articles, this article smacked of vitality and life. Not only was I smitten, I felt refreshed and invigorated. It felt significant somehow. For the rest of the afternoon, the article's intriguing information and images stirred like fresh breezes in the recesses of my mind.

Some months later, in the same journal, I noticed an advertisement for a "pharmacy in the rainforest" healthcare expedition, a professional excursion into the heart of the Amazon rainforest. My decision to go was almost automatic. I felt a current of excitement at the prospect of entering this exotic other world. I was also curious about indigenous healing practices using plant medicines and unusual spiritual techniques, and in the plant origins of new pharmaceuticals. I signed up for the rainforest trip with a group of my colleagues, curious to learn what healing might mean in a non-pharmaceutical based culture.

I didn't realize that a tantalizing article read in the middle of a monotonous workday marked a significant life-change for me, nor that my growing painful disillusionment over the past few years was in fact "just what the doctor ordered." Nor did I know that this trip into the depths of the Peruvian Amazon rainforest would test my sanity to the limits, radically changing my life's direction, and my notions about reality.

CHAPTER 2

INTO
THE GARDEN
OF EDEN

I stood drenched on a dock along the legendary Amazon River, less than four degrees south of the equator, awaiting our boat assignments. We sixty expedition participants would be sent to three different river campsites, north of the town of Iquitos, Peru. The breeze came hot off the river, and every Nordic pore of my body was

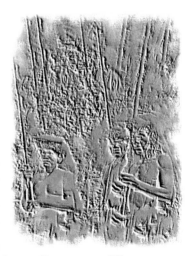

working overtime to generate body-cooling sweat. Minnesota-bred, I was a virtual Eskimo here in the tropics. But no amount of sweat brought relief in this suffocating humidity. One doesn't stay clean or dry in the jungle. There is mud and water everywhere, endless rains (250 days a year), humidity, myriad river waterways, and one's own continuous perspiring.

But I watched the native cargo hands and noticed they were barely sweating at all. Their bodies efficiently conserved precious water. Generations of adaptation had tempered them to the Amazon's heat. I decided this self-drenching, and the water-soaked land squishing its way into my boots, and the daily downpours pummeling the rainforest, were a baptism initiating me into the watery ways of the jungle.

I heard my name called, assigning me to the boat bound for the campsite on the Napo River. The Napo River is one of more than a thousand tributaries feeding the *Rio Amazonas*— the mighty Amazon River—the largest river system in the world. One-fifth of the Earth's fresh water is stored in the Amazon River, with its 14,000 miles of navigable tributaries. I was probably carrying some of it in my canteen at that very moment.

The Amazon River originates from headwaters high in the Andes Mountains of Peru, flows eastward across the South American continent, travels some 4,000 miles, and spills its oceanic abundance into the Atlantic from its mouth in Brazil. In high-water season, the Amazon's mouth can widen to 300 miles, and pour up to 500 billion cubic feet of water into the sea per day. Hard to fathom? Then consider that one day's flow of Amazon waters into the Atlantic would satisfy New York City's fresh water needs for a full nine years!

With a crowd of rickety river taxis, known as *colectivos*, vying for public dock space, we had to board our more modern boat from a private dock. Our 30-foot boat, wooden hull with a palm thatch-roof, had a couple of powerful modern sleek silver Johnson outboard motors hanging out the back of the boat. In contrast, most of the rustic *colectivos* over-flowed with locals and their possessions. Crowds of men, women, and children mingled on the decks of these colorful boats with live chickens, silvery (and smelly!) fish, ripe and rotting bananas, squawking parrots, and various items beyond my ken.

We started down river into the jungle, entering one of the last great wilderness frontiers on Earth. A fishy river breeze blew in my face, and my heart swelled with the sense of high adventure. It was open river as far as I could see. There seemed more water in Peru than land. Here in Iquitos, the Amazon River was five miles wide. The jungle trees on the opposite shore looked one foot tall. I privately dubbed this water-wonderland the "Venice-of-the-Equator."

The Amazon Rainforest covers portions of Brazil, Bolivia, Colombia, Ecuador, Suriname, French Guiana, Venezuela, Guyana, and Peru. Parts of its dense, many-chambered heart are still uncharted, and have yet to be penetrated even by natives. The Peruvian Amazon is homeland of the legendary, single-breasted Amazon warrior women, and the fiercely exotic cat people of the Chavin Cult who took human trophy heads. It is also the place of discovery of a jungle tree whose resilient sap changed the modern world…rubber.

I took one last glance back as the jungle border town of Iquitos vanished around the curve in the Amazon River. No longer able to make out the human forms on the docks, I knew I was leaving civilization behind. I noted the date, October 24, 1994, in my journal. It seemed significant, a mark of passage with deep personal meaning.

Before long, our boat veered to the left, exiting the Amazon onto one of its many tributaries. Now we were heading upstream on the Napo River. The incessant buzzing of the boat's two engines, and the sensations and visual effect of ploughing through a never-ending sea-of-green vegetation, was hypnotic.

Hours passed. Then I noticed the vegetation along the narrowing river's edge was now growing thicker, taller and closer to the banks. Sparsely scattered 20-foot trees gave way to 40-foot *moriche* palms whose tops dotted the tree-skyline. The two walls of green vegetation lining the banks, multiple layers and shades of green upon green, became so dense that no light penetrated them.

As our boat entered deeper into the jungle, the vegetation grew even denser, and its canopy rose on either side of us like canyon walls. Now 60-foot trees were dwarfed by 120-foot *ceiba*, or kapok trees. We were entering the primal rainforest, original growth untouched by man. The jungle now seemed to press upon me with an unnerving, primeval force. The sensation was almost claustrophobic. I was surrounded, and made to feel puny. Vegetation ruled here, with its teeming animal life. And its palpable mystery.

The rainforest is truly the Earth's greatest life-expression, unless you count the seas. It renders insignificant the seven wonders of the world. Now, carried upriver into the deepening jungle, the effect of what I was seeing, the potency of my surroundings, suddenly broke through a protective shield behind which I usually lived unaware. I was literally overwhelmed by a transcendent vision, utterly real and of this world. I was in the midst of the original creation, watching the ultimate masterpiece, Eden itself, unfold before me. In this setting, simply to be alive was larger-than-life.

The trip to our first camp took three hours in our speedy

dual-engine boat. Along the way we passed several *ribereños* settlements along the river's edge. Ribereños are river people of mixed ethnic backgrounds—mainly Spanish, Indian, and African—who live along the river's edge. Though contemporary, their lifestyle is reminiscent of that of their ancestors. They still live in thatched roof huts, the men hunt and fish, and they still use slash-and-burn agricultural techniques to grow food.

As we passed by, the men were casting their fishnets into the river from the bank. The fish they caught would be placed alive in tubs of water—the equivalent of jungle refrigerators—to be killed just before they were eaten.

The women were either busy washing muddy clothes in the river, or tending their many children, while the children played, chasing skinny chickens and each other along the bank and under the raised stilt huts. These ribereños were part of a timeless stream going back for millennia, still living the changeless ways of the rainforest.

I sat mesmerized, watching the river of life go by, being carried along in its currents. How simple and peaceful life was here. I had come home to something deep inside myself. I had fallen into a natural rhythm in me. I hoped it would last.

Hours later, in mellow spirits, we reached the dock of our first camp. Our group of healthcare professionals had come to learn about the medicinal bounty of nature, and to experience the mythic jungle seen only in countless movies. The expedition promised a feast for our senses as well as our professional/scientific intellects.

We jostled excitedly under the thatched roof, grabbed our cameras and backpacks, and stepped off the boat onto dry land. To my amazement, each boat-hand carried more than his own body weight, while I was wilting like a wet leaf from the humidity carrying only my camera. These incredibly fit indigenous held 50-pound provision cases in each hand, while huge bundles of bananas and other accessories hung on their backs by straps across their foreheads.

The river water levels, which fluctuate as much as forty feet throughout the year, were now at low level. To reach our camp we walked half a mile along a narrowing path, straight into the thick, lush, green-darkness of the primal rainforest whose canopy virtually extinguished the sky. The intensity of the vegetation was overwhelming. The deeper we went, the more palpably I sensed the jungle's vastness, its devouring density, its overwhelming power.

The mere factual data of the Amazon rainforest, her bio-chart, so to speak, is astonishing. She contains as much as 50-75% of the Earth's animal and plant species. Her vast vegetation produces a full 20% of the Earth's oxygen, one reason my lungs breathed easier despite the suffocating humidity. Possibly a million plant species comprise this mass of vegetation, of which only 25,000 species have been identified. In this regard, you might say we humans have discovered a needle of the Amazon, while the haystack remains a mystery. One hectare (a little less than 2.5 acres) of tropical rainforest may contain up to 100 different tree species, compared to 10 or 12 tree species in a temperate forest, such as the boundary water forests of the Great Lakes area of my native Minnesota.

The Amazon rainforest's fecund, biotic richness makes her the world's petri dish in many respects, not the least being pharmaceutical. Her rich canopy of tropical vegetation is home to 3,000 bird species, or one-third of the world's bird species. Their constant twittering and chirping now was in itself a dense canopy of sound, rich and deeply soothing. More than 4,000 species of butterflies and 20,000 species of moths flourish here, or roughly a quarter of their respective species found on Earth. It seemed they always fluttered about, solitary or in sudden swarms, flashing hues in the play of shifting jungle shadows.

Besides her rich, colorful fecundity, the rainforest holds secrets that may alter the course of medicine. (Some people say her most potent secrets are even now infiltrating the planetary consciousness, seeding many with the purpose of saving her reverend self.) Her native cultures long ago identified, and use to this day with profound healing effects, numerous medicinal plants we Westerners are still ignorant of. The awareness of this remarkable store of medicinal knowledge had drawn me here with a sense of purpose. Now, on a slow march into her interior, I felt charged with life and knew I had made the right decision to come.

Upon reaching the camp, we quickly turned our small patch of paradise into a loud, chaotic beehive of activity. Three wild macaws, provoked by our group discharge of hyper Western energy, added their screeches of displeasure to the fever pitch. They actually swooped through the camp, down past our ears, wings fluttering and flashing blue/yellow and red/blue streaks. A pair of small saddle-backed tamarin monkeys peeked from around the back of a tree to see what all the commotion was about. Then, as if on cue, they came out and "monkeyed around" for our ready cameras, chasing each other for a few moments before disappearing offstage into the dense green forest from which they came.

It took a couple of hours for all of us—humans and animals—to get used to each other, settle in, and settle down. As a jungle calm returned, heat and humidity exerted an irresistible soporific effect on us *gringos*. Before long, most of us were either dozing off under the mosquito netting in our camp beds, or sitting around in a lethargic stupor.

The camp was surprisingly neat, well-stocked and comfortable, with a palm-thatched roof that was remarkably rainproof, mosquito-netted sleeping quarters situated at one end, and outdoor latrines with showers dispensing river water, at the other. Clean water (bottled in Iquitos) and food were shipped in three times weekly aboard the San Pedro, an old rickety wooden supply boat that made the African Queen look like the Queen Mary, and which made our future provisions seem a risky proposition.

Yet with our needs so well provided for, and our itinerary so neatly arranged, it was easy to be lulled into a sense that all was under control, and that there was no danger in our jungle surroundings.

After lunch, Juan, our native guide, rounded us up for our first official expedition from our camp into the jungle. Juan was a handsome young man in his mid-twenties, with deep brown eyes and an open smile. His slight build belied his intensity. And the glint now in his eyes told me we were about to get our jungle feet wet. So off we went with Juan in the lead.

The purpose of our first jungle trek was to acquaint us with our surroundings before we began our formal ethnobotanical education, our primary reason for coming. Every walk in the jungle plunges one into an infinitude of life that is indescribable. To behold it requires more eyes than are in one head, and more attention than we tend to use in ordinary life. Every moment had something to offer. One moment I'd be swatting at swarms of hungry mosquitoes, the next I'd look up to see several iridescent hummingbirds flashing metallic red, blue, and green, darting and sucking sweet nectar from the yellow blooms of a wild mango tree.

A short distance from the camp, Juan stopped and pointed at a spot near the base of a tree. Using a stick, he uncovered a hole and teased out a six-inch long brown hairy tarantula, assuring us this variety wasn't poisonous to humans. Still, I instinctively stepped back and nearly squashed a battalion of leafcutter ants marching behind me across the path, transporting pieces of foraged leaves and petals back to their colony. It was an impressive sight to see several thousand quarter-inch leafcutter ants carrying half-inch pieces of green jungle on their backs. I leaned against a nearby tree and aimed my camera to capture the scene. Suddenly Juan shouted at me to get off the tree immediately! It was a *tangarana* tree, explained Juan. When touched, it unleashes multitudes of ferocious biting ants that it houses for its own protection. I immediately recoiled from this incredible "tree that bites," thankful for the warning.

"Look over here," said Juan pointing his stick. Looking down, I saw the most striking little creature I'd ever seen— a jet black frog with brilliant red mottling, less than an inch long, hopping amidst the leaf-litter, so perfectly designed it looked like a little plastic child's toy. Camera ready, I went in for a close-up shot of this stunning little frog. When he began to hop out of camera range, I reached down intending to manually adjust his position, eliciting yet another warning shout from Juan.

"*Don't touch!* It's a poison arrow frog."

Juan explained how the frog's skin secreted a potentially

lethal toxin which natives used to tip their poison darts and arrows. Lordy! Talk about unwary neophytes! Five minutes into my first official trek and I'd almost assaulted an army of ants, been bitten by a tree, and killed myself with the cutest little frog I'd ever seen! Now I was afraid to turn around without detailed instructions.

I was learning the local fact of life, gospel to every native: The jungle is a vast, teeming, unpredictable place, much of it stunningly beautiful, and some of it absolutely deadly. It is a place of contrasts and absurd paradoxes, where all is not as it seems. Here one cannot naïvely trust one's impressions, a fact that, when it sinks in, is both sobering and disorienting. Here scary hairy tarantulas are safe to handle; adorable miniature toy-frogs are lethal to touch; and if you lean against the wrong tree, it will bite you! By the end of that first day I felt a bit like Alice in the Heart of Darkness.

Come bedtime I was exhausted, sensorily overwhelmed, and ready to sleep. Yet as I drifted off, I had the sense that a day in the jungle with my eyes wide open was as surreal as any dream I might have while asleep.

The next morning we visited one of the Yagua Indian tribes who still thrive along the Napo River. The Yaguas, according to their creation myth, believe they once lived in the sky. But having depleted the sky-game that sustained them, the tribe, out of necessity, lowered a brother and sister to the Earth. So the first Yagua came to Earth. Once there, the brother and sister experienced their first storm, with torrential rains, earth-shaking thunder, and a roaring wind. In the midst of the storm, a gigantic tree fell to the ground. Its heavy trunk sank deep into the earth and became a torrent of water that we now call the Amazon River. The tree's branches changed into the Amazon's numerous tributaries. Its many fallen leaves became an abundance of river fish. Wood chunks from its trunk were transformed into large canoes which filled with Yagua and other Indian tribes. So, according to Yagua legend, the Amazon was formed and the Earth was populated.

A pleasant boat ride down and across the Yanamono River separated our camp from the Yagua tribe. As we neared their village I saw a greeting committee straight out of National Geographic magazine—six Yagua men and two Yagua women standing at the river's edge patiently awaiting our arrival. The men wore skirts of shredded thatchlike fibers— somewhat like rough stringy floor-mop—and elaborate woven palm headgear that looked like ornate Amazonian Easter bonnets. All fibers were made of *chambira* palm shoots. The women wore colorful wrap-around cotton skirts. Except for the shredded palm-fiber "bibs" that hung over the women's chest and back, both men and women were bare-breasted. Their bodies and faces were painted with patches and patterns of orange-red *achiote* and black *huito* plant dyes.

I was a bit taken aback by the 10-foot poison dart blowguns, the *pucunas*, each of the Yagua men sported. And I felt a bit more at ease when a dozen more shy Yagua women showed up, two with babies on their hips. When Juan began speaking with them, their gentle smiles allayed my remaining fears about ferocious jungle warriors.

Next they cheerfully led us into their village a hundred yards away and took us into their *cocamera*, a large oval-shaped communal dwelling whose palm-thatched dome roof sloped all the way to the ground. There were no partition walls inside; the family compartments were separated only by floor mats. The only furniture in this completely open space were log stools and hammocks. On the surrounding inner walls of this traditional communal house and ceremonial center were hung their native crafts—various fiber arts, wooden animal carvings, and colorful beadwork—their *artesanía*, as they call it.

While we were there, a young Yagua girl demonstrated the spinning technique used to produce cordage for hammocks, fishing lines, nets, and bags. Rolling a small flat band of *Astrocaryum* palm fibers across her thigh, she produced a single-ply cord. Two- or three-ply cord is used for items requiring more strength such as net bags, hammocks, and baskets. And the Yagua use *capinurí* tree fibers to make the fiber-cloth mats which serve as their only floor covering.

Glancing around the communal hut I noticed simple drinking vessels made of *calabash* gourd, and wooden troughs and rockers used for preparing food. Then a young Yagua chief-in-training stepped forward to tell us more about their life in the jungle. The Yagua's agricultural diet is predominately sweet, like their natures. Their staple crop is sweet manioc, supplemented with maize, yams, bananas, sweet potatoes, sugar cane, papaya, and pineapple. This high natural sugar diet probably explains why most of the elders had lost most of their teeth.

Of course the Yagua regularly eat fish, and sometimes meat. The handsome young Yagua chief-in-training proudly informed us that their game included deer, tapir, monkey, agouti, anteater, sloth, armadillo, and river turtle. The arrows, spears, and blowgun darts they hunted with were often tipped with poison extracted either from frog venom, or from the poisonous curare plant which is also the source of the pharmaceutical drug tubocurarine.

"Curare" comes from an Indian word meaning, "bird" and "to kill." The active compounds contained in its bark are laboriously extracted and filtered into a dark liquid that is heated, cooled, and reheated until it becomes a thick, viscous syrup. The tips of arrows, darts, and spears are dipped and rolled in this tarry substance, then set by a fire to dry and harden. When a strong dose of curare poison penetrates an animal's flesh, it slows the animal down, making it easy to catch. Eventually, it paralyzes the animal's diaphragm muscles, causing it to stop breathing and die.

After the formal presentations to our group were finished, an eager five year old Yagua boy took us outside to see his family's garden. When we asked him if it contained any medicinal plants, he pointed out, amongst the manioc, sugar cane, and rice shoots, random plantings of ginger, *curarina*, and *paico*. To our amazement, he not only told us their Yagua names (Juan served as his translator) but also rattled off their medicinal properties.

"Curarina we use for snake bites, and paico for worms," he recited. "And ginger is good for bronchitis, headaches, stomach problems, and rheumatism."

Not only were the names on the tip of his tongue, this five year old knew how to use these medicinal plants in his family's front yard "medicine cabinet."

The rainforest provided for the Yagua's every need. Its plant-life was a universal currency bent to every conceivable use by their inventive minds. It gave them food, medicine, clothing, furniture, poisons, paints, dyes, housing, and a wealth of other utilitarian and decorative items.

In person, these native peoples seemed less primitive than I'd been taught to assume. In their presence, the word "primitive" had an unpleasant ideological ring. The phrase "of the earth" seemed more fittingly honorable, for the Yagua seemed intimately connected to the earth in a way that I wished I could be.

After our visit we walked back to the boat. On our way we passed a small black water lagoon surrounded by several water oxen. Dozens of gigantic *Victoria regias*, or Amazon water lilies, floated on its surface amidst beds of water lettuce, their huge round flat green leaves spanning from three to six feet in diameter. We saw one mother caringly washing her baby on a large lily leaf, nature's bassinet. Had Courier and Ives painted a jungle greeting card, this would have been the scene.

On the third morning, somewhat acclimatized to this forbidding and exotic new environment, we began our group's field-workshop on the ethnobotanical origins of pharmaceuticals. We gathered under the canopy-shade of an *Inga* tree, commonly called an "ice cream bean tree," to hear Western scientists teach us the history of jungle pharmacy.

Charles, a gray-bearded American Ph.D. botanist and expert on rainforest medicinal plants and foods, was our first instructor. He was clearly at home in the jungle, being the only one besides Juan wearing Bermuda shorts. The rest of us were still over-dressed for protection. Charles began by asking Juan to chop down several fruits—they looked like thick two-foot long green beans—from the Inga tree with his machete. Juan quickly obliged. His expertise with the machete was impressive; it seemed as if a metallic extension of his arm.

We were each given a piece of the pod-like fruit, which we cracked open. Inside we found large seeds coated with white pulp, which Charles encouraged us to eat. We sucked the sweet meaty pulp off the seeds with greedy slurps. Mmmm...ice cream bean, a non-frozen tropical ice cream treat!

Charles then explained the Inga tree's many medicinal uses. "Its white fruit-pulp is used to wipe the eyes and clean the teeth. Its bark and seeds are used to treat children with dysentery, a common ailment in the tropics." Charles paused a moment to enjoy the fruits of his own lecture, sucking like the rest of us on his ice cream bean. Then he wiped his beard and commented, "Medicine never tasted so good!"

With this simple demonstration, Charles pointed out the most basic and intriguing aspect of the indigenous people's relationship to the sea of vegetation in which they live and thrive: Plants are primary life-givers as food and medicine. You might say they make no rigid distinction between the food and medicinal uses of plants; they recognize food as medicine, and medicine as food.

This indigenous perspective is now taking hold in the West, where scientists are beginning to study certain foods that may potentially have medicinal value. Western medicine is beginning to place foods that heal into categories, such as nutraceuticals and functional foods. Some of our most popular foods are now recognized as powerful herbal medicines, such as ginger and garlic. Charles pointed out that by studying which rainforest food/plants the indigenous use as medicines, we may make important new drug discoveries that could benefit mankind.

Biome – "A community of living organisms." American Heritage Dictionary.

Charles finished his presentation as we were sucking the last bits of sweet meat of the last of our ice cream beans. The next lecturer was Eric, an American ethnobotanist with extensive Central and South American rainforest experience, who had worked with dozens of shamans over the years. Clearly a man with jungle-savvy, physically fit and in the prime of his career, he came down the trail and joined our group with a machete tucked in his belt. It looked like it belonged there. He introduced himself to our group and told us to prepare to hike deeper into the jungle. There a passionate ethnobotanist is most at home, walking and talking about plant medicines. As we rose and prepared to march, Eric began his lecture.

"Tropical rainforests, containing the richest biomes on Earth, represent a vast self-replenishing store of natural resources. For eons, by virtue of their bio-richness, rainforests have contributed myriad plant, animal, mineral, pharmaceutical, and other treasures (not to mention oxygen) of great significance to the Earth's survival and well being. Let's consider various local plants and their current and potential medicinal/pharmaceutical value. This consideration is the very heart and soul of ethnobotany."

We started down the jungle trail with Eric in the lead. Ethnobotany—"ethno" from ethnic, and "botany" for plant—is the scientific study of plants used by native peoples. A key aim of ethnobotany is to determine which plants the indigenous use as folk medicines have active chemical constituents of medicinal value. The goal is to discover new medicines and pharmaceuticals that can cure human ills and relieve human suffering.

Many ethnobotanists and other scientists believe the plant kingdom may hold keys for cures to such modern ills as AIDS, cancer, and a host of other diseases that have historically plagued mankind. Modern botanical medicine success stories have bolstered these hopes. The drug Taxol, extracted from the Pacific yew tree found in the American Northwest, has proven effective in treating ovarian and metastatic breast cancers. The Indians of that area have long used the yew tree for a variety of medicinal purposes. The rosy periwinkle of Madagascar, now found also in Central and South America, has given us vincristine and vinblastine, used to treat childhood leukemia and Hodgkin's disease.

Amazonian plants and trees have yielded important modern medicines such as tubocurarine and quinine. Quinine signaled the end of the malarial scourge in many mosquito-infested parts of the world. The threat of malaria made the bitter-tasting gin and tonic (quinine water), the British drink of choice in colonial India and throughout the tropics.

As he walked, Eric delivered a fascinating lecture that was a blend of botany, medical history, and interesting anecdotes. At one point he stopped before a sizeable tree branch that had fallen onto the path. He quickly drew his machete from his belt and used it to point out a vine of green, heart-shaped leaves two inches long wrapped around the branch.

"This leaf," he said, "can either kill you or help cure you. Anyone know what it is?" Whoa, powerful little green leaf, I thought. There were no guesses from the group. "I'll give you a clue," Eric continued. "It's used both by indigenous hunters in Amazonia, and by surgeons in modern hospitals."

We should have guessed, but we didn't. We gathered closer around to Eric to look at this important specimen. It turned out to be the curare vine we had learned about only yesterday at the Yagua village, the one they used to make the poison with which they tipped their arrows. Now here was the devastating little leaf in person, which is also the source of the pharmaceutical tubocurarine.

Most surgeries in the last century have benefited from this potent drug. A powerful muscle relaxant, it decreases the amount of anesthesia required for surgery, thus lessening negative side effects and associated risks. And it makes possible delicate operations where total muscle relaxation is essential.

Scientists and ethnobotanists conceived the surgical uses of curare after watching its disabling effects on animals hit with curare poison-tipped arrows. When used in small enough doses, it immobilizes the human body without stopping the heart. Every modern operating room relies on Amazonian tubocurarine for successful surgeries.

Yet curare is so slow-growing it has never been cultivated for medicine. And its intensive exploitation for medicinal use over the past eighty years, and increasing rainforest devastation, is causing concern over curare's availability in the future. Having dispensed thousands of vials of tubocurarine to operating rooms in my career, I can't imagine what will replace it if it disappears.

These are but a few of the half a hundred examples of the rainforest's contribution to modern medicine. Now consider that to date, less than half of 1% of all plant species have been studied for their pharmaceutical/medicinal value. And as the rainforests contain the widest and most potent variety of plant species on Earth, it was inevitable that modern ethnobotanists would finally come to learn from their rainforest counterparts, the jungle shamans who have long been studying, experimenting with, and using medicinal plants to heal.

Over centuries of experimentation and practice, native

shamans have discovered, categorized and harnessed both the medicinal and toxic properties of innumerable plants, many still unknown to modern Western medicine. These shamans have transmitted their unique body of knowledge through long and arduous apprenticeships—shamanic equivalents of medical degrees. And we in the West are now beginning to recognize the value of centuries of accumulated shamanic medicinal wisdom.

As dinnertime approached, I was covered with the usual sticky layer of salty sweat, and eager to return to camp for one of my three or four daily showers. Our only relief from the sweltering heat was the cool river water, piped into a wooden shower stall and through a showerhead (I suspect it was also a fish-filter). That our showers left us smelling a bit fishy already seemed moot. "Fishy" was just one ingredient that, mixed with "sweat," "mold," "mildew," and other unidentifiable jungle odors, created a unique and persistent aroma I called "eau de tropical." It became the resident joke.

Dinner consisted of grilled *paiche* fish (which can grow to several hundred pounds in Amazon's wider expanses), fresh *chonta* salad (made from heart of a palm tree), nutritious *camu camu* fruit juice (more vitamin C than any other fruit), roasted yuca roots, and sweet succulent papayas. After dinner we were introduced to don Francisco, an Iquitos shaman ritually dressed in an earth-toned short tunic and matching headband trimmed with black geometric patterns. When he offered to perform tobacco healings for any who were interested, I grabbed my camera like an excited tourist and followed him down the path, babbling to my colleagues about how "cool" this was. I was eager to get some "I saw a real shaman" snap shots for my Amazon rainforest photo album. I had no idea what I was getting myself into.

Don Francisco led us to an area by a small hut, and we sat on the ground before him. He lit a hand-rolled cigarette and began alternately whistling a haunting tune, and blowing billowing puffs of smoke at our gathering. Our camera flashes popped and we watched him with great interest, as if he were an exotic local nightclub act.

Then he offered to perform private healings in the small hut. I got up and went to stand in line with the others. I intended to get the most bang for my expedition buck, and maybe another picture—me with a real shaman—for my album. I had no clue what I was waiting for, or what healing I might need, or even what a shaman really was. It just seemed like harmless fun. I admit with some embarrassment that I approached the event in a spirit not far removed from having my picture taken with Santa at a local mall.

While waiting in line, I talked and laughed too loudly, and a bit nervously. Then I looked up to find myself two people away from the door. Now my attention was drawn to the shaman's hut. I grew silent and felt an odd stirring in my gut, some kind of force or energy. Oddly, I seemed to "feel" what was going on inside the hut. I had no idea what don Francisco was doing, but I sensed some sort of power in there. Suddenly I felt like a child about to enter a haunted Halloween house. I didn't know what to expect, and I was afraid to go in.

Then my turn came. I set my camera on the ground outside the hut and went in. It was dark and smoky inside. I saw don Francisco, or rather his form, standing in a cloud of smoke. He motioned for me to sit on the small wooden stool in front of him. He lit another hand-rolled cigarette and unimpressively proceeded to whistle his song and blow smoke over me. *This, is a healing?* I thought. Nothing was happening.

Two minutes later, everything changed. My body began to shake and my head arched back. When don Francisco stopped, so did the shaking, and my body returned to normal. When he started up, my body began to shake and arch again. After four or five of these stops and starts, he was finished. I was utterly disoriented and glad it was over. I couldn't explain what had happened. Maybe it's a placebo reaction, I thought. Only I didn't believe in shamans!

I got up from the stool and walked out of the hut. I was no longer a glib, laughing tourist. I was a bewildered woman trying to sort out what had happened to me, or what, if anything, had been done to me. The others were still waiting in line for their healings. Then I bent down to pick up my camera, completely lost control of my body, fell to the ground and lay there, shaking violently. I was infused with some kind of energy that my body didn't know what to do with. Several pharmacists rushed over to me, thinking I was having a seizure, a heart attack, or a diabetic reaction. The same fearful thoughts occurred to me as I was shaking. Yet another part of me sensed that this was something different.

Then don Francisco came rushing out of the hut and began to press certain spots around my neck. Soon the shaking stopped. He spoke in Spanish, and someone translated.

"She has a block in her neck."

I had no idea what he meant. It wasn't a medical phrase I had ever heard. There was nothing wrong with my neck as far as I knew. I didn't think to ask him what he meant. Later on I would wish I had. Don Francisco helped me to stand up. I felt more or less in control of my body again. I didn't know what had come over me.

The next morning I still felt shaky and my perceptions

seemed altered. In fact, I was more perceptive than usual. Colors appeared more vivid, the edges of things were sharper. While walking at the edge of the camp, the distinct white markings on the faces of two Titi monkeys hiding 60 feet up in the trees caught my eye. Yesterday the jungle was a monotonous blur of a few shades of green fading into each other. Today it was a rich, multi-layered tapestry woven of many distinct shades of green, brown, lights, shadows, and the random vivid flashes of exotic flora and fauna.

Even my sense of smell was heightened. Aromas flooded my nose. I smelled morning eggs cooking 100 yards away, mixed with earthy, pungent rainforest odors and my artificially perfumed soap. This is a dog's view of life, I thought…all nose. Or was this what life was *really* like when one was open to it. Yet I felt too open…anxious, vulnerable, newborn.

Who *are* these shamans, I wondered. What actually happened last night? I checked in with a few others who'd had healings, but no one shared my experience. I felt like I was babbling. So I kept quiet and ate my breakfast.

The morning lecture was just what I needed. It got me back into my head, and my hypersensitivity faded into the background. Afterwards, we started off on a long trek into the primary rainforest. "Primary" rainforest is a botanical term that denotes original, unfelled forest growth. Engulfed in the dense green mosaic, our group soon fell silent. The rhythmic movements of my own walking, and the intense vegetative energy, somehow put me back into the sensitive state I had managed to suppress during the lecture.

It was a fascinating day. We explored a variety of leaves, trees, roots, and vines, all containing pharmaceutical ingredients used by jungle shamans and Western physicians. The more time I spent in the jungle, the more I wondered how, out of a possible million plant species in the Amazon, had shamans identified so many with such potent healing, or deadly, or mind-altering characteristics? How many more botanical treasures remained to be discovered—or might never be discovered—hidden in this green oceanic mass?

I was still not myself by the time we returned to camp at the end of the day. As dusk fell, the shifting jungle shadows played on my imagination and my heightened senses. I had the eerie impression that I was somehow connected to, and in some strange way infiltrated by, the surrounding vegetation. The jungle and all around me was softening, and I was merging with it. The boundaries between me and the plant kingdom were melting. I had the sense that the jungle had a soul. But I wasn't even sure if I had one.

Fearing the shaman had done something to me, I decided to talk to our ethnobotanist, Eric. Eric had mentioned working with many shamans, and I thought he might be able to shed some light on what I was feeling. I cornered him after dinner and told him something of my dilemma. He listened to my story with a receptive ear.

"I'll introduce you to a more powerful shaman tomorrow after our workshop," he said when I'd finished. "His name is don Antonio. He may be able to help."

The next morning we were scheduled to take another long hike into the rainforest with Eric and Charles to meet the shaman don Antonio. Before leaving, Eric gave a fascinating lecture on the nature of shamans and their unique work with jungle medicines. He explained that a rainforest shaman's healing practices are a blend of both plant medicine and spirit invocation. Jungle shamans, he said, have an intimate and mysterious relationship with both plants and with heal-ing spirits whom they regard as significant intermediaries in the healing process. And in their healing rituals, they ad-minister plant medicines, and summon these spirits on behalf of the patient. They regard both "agencies" as necessary to fully transfer the healing energies to the patient.

Eric explained that shamans are the keepers of the pre-cious knowledge of rainforest plants, and that it is important, even for us in the West, to conserve their priceless oral tradi-tion of plant lore, acquired over centuries and passed on over generations. Every time a shaman dies, a library is burned down. And every time a rainforest is felled, a pharmacy is destroyed.

Eric led our group into the jungle and we started down a winding path. As we walked, he continued his lecture, tell-ing us the story behind Western medicine's disconnection from its botanical origins. Before scientific advances in labo-ratory synthesis of new compounds, the plant kingdom was mankind's primary source of medicine, Eric said. A dramatic change occurred in the 1930s, with the advent of synthetic chemistry. By the 1970s, science had achieved stunning suc-cesses in synthesizing blockbuster drugs such as Tagamet and Valium and a host of other pharmaceutical wonders.

It was now cheaper and easier to chemically invent new compounds in a laboratory than to send teams of experts into the jungles, randomly seeking new medicinal plants buried amongst a near-million possible candidates. In addition, there is the expense of testing those few promising candi-dates that might be found, and finally turning some of these into reliable medicinal compounds. Not surprisingly, the pharmaceutical industry quickly lost interest in plants as sources of potential new medicines.

In the new era of wonder drugs, science seemed to have rendered nature's medicinal offerings obsolete. Growing disenchantment with the liabilities and side-effects of modern drugs; plus new techniques for purifying, analyzing, and assaying plant samples; and a growing, grudging respect for the body of medicinal knowledge accumulated over centuries by jungle shamans have now rekindled strong interest in the rainforest as a source of potent new medicines. As Eric ironically noted, the very science that had once taken researchers like himself out of the jungle, was now sending them back in again, in some cases making them almost virtual shamanic apprentices.

We came to a small stream and followed the small path that ran alongside it, deep in the jungle. It finally led us out into a clearing where we saw a tiny, thatched-roof hut, perhaps eight by eight feet. This was the home of shaman don Antonio Montero Pisco, spiritually descended from a long lineage of shamans of the Cocama tribe. I could hardly imagine a more isolated spot to live.

At our approach, a humble-looking indigenous man came from inside the hut and stood in the doorway, calmly looking out at us. Eric approached him, and politely began to speak with him in Spanish. Eric then turned around to introduce our group to shaman don Antonio.

His appearance was a bit of a surprise. He wore no shaman's garb like don Francisco, and no woven fiber garb like the Yagua. Instead, he wore a faded T-shirt, a ragged pair of Western pants, no shoes, a machete casually dangled from his right arm. He looked much like any of the hired locals who helped around the lodge. This is a shaman, I thought? He looked absolutely down to earth, and of the earth, too.

I didn't have time to think about it. Don Antonio came out of his doorway and started down a jungle path. I stepped quickly in line behind him and we were off, following him single file into the jungle. As we walked, I looked down at his bare, thickly calloused feet sticking out of his hand-me-down Western pants. Charles, walking right behind me, called out in Spanish to don Antonio,

"No *zapatos* (shoes), don Antonio?"

Don Antonio, pointing at his bare feet, said something back that made Charles laugh.

"Don Antonio says his are the best shoes of all," Charles translated for us.

Don Antonio then surged sure-footedly ahead of the group, moving with ease and familiarity, as if the soles of his feet knew every inch of the jungle floor. At times his toes gripped the muddy earth with a squishing sound.

I was suddenly struck by the absurd contrast between our product-burdened group, outfitted in slick-modern jungle attire, and this humble shaman whose three-piece outfit consisted of an old T-shirt, a tattered pair of pants, and a machete. We had almost enough gear to cross a continent, climb Mt. Everest and land on the moon—canteens, rain hats, compasses, flashlights, sunglasses, backpacks, hip packs, bug spray, water-proof watches, over-the-ankle hiking boots, the latest high-tech cameras and binoculars, and more—every product the best camping/safari stores could sell us as insurance against our worst fears.

Until now, I'd imagined we looked dashing, like a pack of Indiana Joneses. Now I chuckled at how ridiculous we must have looked to don Antonio. We were wary jungle tres-passers functioning under the premise that we needed maximum protection *from* nature, while don Antonio was a welcome inhabitant walking at ease in his backyard. We were out of our element, strangers to nature; he was *in* his element and at home in nature.

After a while, he stopped and pointed to a woody liana, a vine clinging to a tree by curved, claw-like spines extending from its leaves. *"Es medicina,"* he said. It's medicine. Charles told us the vine, aptly named, was *uña de gato*, or cat's claw, an herbal remedy used in the United States for a variety of inflammatory and immune-related problems. National Cancer Institute research, he added, has verified some of the immunostimulant and anticancer properties of cat's claw.

Don Antonio then explained, with Eric translating, that he used cat's claw often in his healing practice to treat conditions ranging from ulcers, cancer, and arthritis to various other forms of inflammatory conditions. With Eric questioning, don Antonio further explained that the healing spirit of cat's claw is a big powerful black monkey. "Each medicinal plant," don Antonio went on to explain, "has its own spirit form that does the healing." As he looked into our bewildered eyes, don Antonio added, "That is how it is." While I had no reason to believe that what he'd just told us was true, I must admit I was intrigued by the fact that the indigenous uses of this plant closely match Western scientific appraisals of its healing properties.

Don Antonio started off again, moving briskly down the sodden jungle path. In his company I felt recharged and inspired to learn more, and I now kept up with him more easily. A mysterious dimension of healing seemed palpable in this unassuming middle-aged Cocama healer. It kindled a kind of spark in me. In my vulnerable state, I matched his footsteps, step for step. I may have regarded him a bit like the duckling who believes the first creature she sees after emerging from the egg is her mother. But I could see from the way my comrades also regarded him that there was something remarkable about don Antonio. He seemed to embody priceless knowledge that Western medicine had both lost and never learned.

Now don Antonio stopped in front of another tree, drew his machete, and with one quick, deft stroke, cut into its smooth greenish-white bark. Then he quietly waited, staring at the incision. Within a few seconds, a red resin bled from the wound.

"*Sangre de grado*," don Antonio said.

"Dragon's blood," Eric translated. Don Antonio wiped some of the red sap from the tree and rubbed it vigorously on the back of his hand till it formed a white paste. He told us that he used sangre de grado orally to treat diarrhea, and topically to heal wounds, that it both stops bleeding and disinfects the wound.

"It's the rainforest's mercurochrome," said Charles, adding that scientific research on sangre de grado had shown it to be effective in treating a variety of ailments. The proanthocycanidins extracted from this sap are currently being used in wound-healing, anti-viral and anti-inflammatory medications, and to treat Herpes simplex and infectious diarrhea. Various other applications are also being tested. Another case of modern science validating traditional indigenous plant medicines. What else do they know that we don't know, I wondered?

With every new detail of this afternoon's lecture, don Antonio, a diminutive, unassuming Cocama man gained stature in my eyes. I watched him, standing calmly, his machete tucked in his belt and the back of his hand covered with a smear of white paste which had healed and perhaps saved the lives of his distant ancestors. He was like some rainforest Yoda. I wondered how many medicinal secrets, stored in the library of his mind, which might prove equally useful to the West.

By the end of the day I was completely under his spell. When we arrived back at don Antonio's hut, the group lined up to thank him. Eric pulled me to the back of the line so that I could have a private moment with the shaman at the end. Finally, I was the only one left.

Through my tears, I told don Antonio about don Francisco's healing, and of the disturbing shaking, and the strange shift in perception that was still occurring. I told him how uneasy I was with this, and that it made me fear for my sanity. It all came out in a torrent. I even told him of my mother's episode in the mental hospital, of my disillusionment with my career and with modern pharmacy. In short, I completely lost it. I was sobbing by the end. Don Antonio kindly listened to it all, patiently observing me, calmly present.

When I was finished, he simply said, "You have enough energy to be a shaman yourself."

I responded with another flood of tears. "You don't understand. My problem is my job. And I'm afraid I may be going crazy."

"You asked me, and I told you," he quietly answered, his expression unchanging.

That was all he said. I didn't feel a bit better. I wondered why I'd even bothered to reveal my deepest feelings to him. As far as I could see he hadn't helped me a bit, and had in fact only added to my confusion. I wanted him to put the cap back on the bottle, to put an end to the process the first shaman seemed to have started. I had also wanted him to give me "the answer" to my worldly career crisis, and to banish my fears. Weren't shamans, like magicians, supposed to have unusual powers? I decided this idea was nonsense, pure mythology.

Yet all the way back through the jungle to the camp, I couldn't get don Antonio's face out of my mind.

CHAPTER 3

LOSING MY
MIND...COMING
TO MY SENSES

T he next phase started the night of our departure from the camp. There was a farewell party after dinner, complete with native music...flutes, drums, maracas, even a strumming guitar, and lots of bad yet enthusiastic singing. Some of the native tour guides with secret dreams of being pop stars in the States played several songs by Santana they'd learned from the radio.

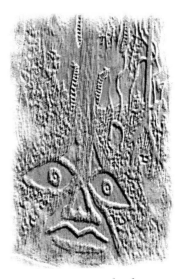

I could tell I was going to miss the rainforest, its rhythms, textures, fragrances and sounds; rising at dawn to the earthy sweet smell of *copal* tree resin, the stunning cobalt blue

Morpho size-of-your-open-hand butterflies, and the cease-less chatter of hungry Capuchin monkeys; and the erotic fragrance of the literally intoxicating datura flowers that ex-uded their aroma only after nightfall. Lunch at home would be bland after eating sweet, perfumy, jungle-ripe mangos, meaty agouti stew, and fresh fire-fried piranha river fish be-fore wandering the living green tunnel-like trails with shaman don Antonio as our guide. California evenings would seem incomplete without the distinctive "wolf-whistle" calls of the pauraque, of the nightjar bird family, provocatively calling to his mate after nightfall. And above all I would miss the ceaseless, distant murmuring presence of the Amazon River itself.

I imagine my celebrating pharmacy comrades felt the same. I could see the hot jungle night, the wild music and dancing, and the fiery *aguardiente*, a potent local sugar cane rum, gradually loosening bodies and unleashing passions. There promised to be more than just dancing on this final night. The fecundity of the rainforest is inherently sensual and intoxicating. Its influence can awaken primal instincts and passions even in mild-mannered Western tourists. And tonight, our group had definitely "gone native."

Everyone but me had decided to stay up until our 2 A.M. departure by riverboat back to Iquitos. I definitely felt the electrical charge in the air of those unbelievably potent "Amazon jungle pheromones." By sheer sobriety, I didn't imbibe in the aguardiente, and inherited Scandinavian sto-icism, I held out against the undeniable exotic charms of the last jungle night and our native guides—to which some of the other gals were about to succumb. But I was about to discover how utterly I had succumbed to the exotic power of the jungle itself.

I toured the party scene just long enough to say my last good-byes to the new friends I had made, and would soon be leaving behind forever. Unforgettable as this experience had been for me, I didn't plan on ever returning to Peru. It would be a once-in-a-lifetime experience, to be treasured as a memory.

It was after 9 P.M. when I entered my tent to pack and change clothes for the long up-river boat ride and return flight home. I completed my packing and lay down on the mattress under my mosquito net to reflect upon my trip here. I left the kerosene lamp on, as I had no intention of sleeping. Then I closed my eyes. Suddenly, I found myself walking along a path through the dense jungle in mid-day. The sunlight, shattered by a dense canopy of thick treetops, came through in rays and glimmers, spattering the surrounding foliage with speckled patches of gold. With a start, I opened my eyes. I was back in my tent under my mosquito net, the kerosene lamp glowing.

I blinked a few times, shaken and disoriented by what had seemed a vivid dream. Only I had not fallen asleep. When I closed my eyes again, the same thing happened. Instantly, I found myself in the jungle, still in daylight, walking along a winding path through thick vegetation. More than a mere mental image, I experienced all the physical and sensory impressions of an actual jungle excursion. I had somehow walked through the emerald door and into another jungle reality.

As I walked along a slippery-wet, red clay path thickly littered with damp fallen leaves, my shoulders brushed against the thickly dangling lianas, the "Tarzan vines" that hung from the trees. I was alone, hearing the cacophony of animals and birds, shrouded by dense vegetation, feeling that stiflingly hot Amazon humidity that makes it seem as if you're re-breathing your own hot breath. Once more I opened my eyes and found myself back in the tent, lying on my mattress, the lamp glowing and the jungle outside blanketed in utter darkness.

Both experiences seemed equally real. A blink of my eyes sent me back and forth between two realities, between day and night. The experience was fascinating and unnerving. I would never dare to walk alone into the jungle, which held many dangers. Doing so now, with my eyes closed, I felt in danger of being engulfed…by what I did not know. I felt alone in a primal vastness.

The experience continued for hours. I couldn't leave my eyes closed for long. But when I opened them, I felt drawn back in spite of myself to this inner jungle. I told myself it must be due to exhaustion, a psychological effect of over-stimulation, the sensory overload of new impressions. When I couldn't make it stop, I tried to shrug it off. But it continued for the two more nights, awake and asleep, as we slowly moved upriver toward Iquitos, and from there, out of Peru.

I caught a direct Peru-to-U.S. flight from Iquitos straight to Miami, and passed through Customs beneath disconcertingly bright artificial lights. I felt out of place moving through the airport's modern interior, assaulted by its chemical sterility, the oil-fried odors of the fast-food stands, and the cheap artificial fragrances emanating from the duty-free shops I passed.

Something of the primal jungle had deeply penetrated my psyche. After my baptismal immersion in Amazon Eden, America's technological and commercial opulence seemed hollow, lacking some vital nourishment that I found I now craved. Here I could buy whatever I wanted (or rather could afford). But I felt cut off from the natural order of life. Here my soul was not fed, whereas in the rainforest I was fed on every level without even taking a bite.

Lyrics came to mind from an old popular song about American tourists: *How are ya gonna keep 'em down on the farm, once they've seen Par-ee?* But for me it was Peru. I had the strange impression that my body was on its way back to the farm, but my soul was still somewhere in the Amazon jungle.

For two days after my return, the unusual internal experiences continued. It was more than reverse culture shock. Eyes open or shut, I seemed to live in a state of hyper-awareness. I felt excessive energy and was unable to sleep normally. When I did close my eyes I was instantly back in the Amazon, walking the jungle paths in that strange waking lucid-dream. This state persisted even during sleep so that I seemed to get no rest. It was disorienting and unnerving. I wanted my old life and my old self back. But I didn't know where they had gone.

I was sorry I'd ever met a shaman, if this was his doing. Yet I had an odd sense that the jungle itself was calling me, a vast conscious entity that knew who I was and how to find me. Even in my altered state the idea seemed clearly delusional, a step away from, *"Hello, Amazon Jungle, calling collect for Connie Grauds. Will you accept the charges?"* For the first time in my life, I had good reason to fear for my sanity. And the random energy surges coming on like volcanic eruptions, often at night when I was trying to sleep, didn't help.

Nothing in my Midwest upbringing had prepared me for

this. I'm a sorority sister girl-next-door type, voted Honors Society, Class President, and Outstanding Senior Woman. In my commitment to normalcy I had even abstained from the "sex, drugs, and rock'n'roll" Sixties. I not only didn't inhale, I never showed up at the party. Ironic, given my career in pharmaceuticals. Now I was living in a prolonged altered state. And the only context I had for the experience was my mother's psychosis. Nor could I confide in my equally square circle of friends and colleagues. Thank God my husband, Dean, believed that I wasn't crazy. He provided a safe container for my unfolding experiences, for which I am eternally grateful.

My mind kept fearfully returning to my mother's craziness. I still had vague memories and disturbing impressions of her, both before and after her stint in the mental hospital when I was three years old. She had told me years later how terrified she had been whenever the lights of the loony bin dimmed, knowing someone was getting their shock treatment. She knew they'd come for her sooner or later. And she'd wait in terror for the sound of the orderlies' footsteps coming down the hall…and for her door to open.

She had possessed such a brilliant, creative mind, so much potential. But all her gifts had been channeled into an exotic and unpredictable internal world…one which the doctors had convinced her, and the rest of us, was crazy. And if she wasn't crazy before her medical intervention, she was certainly crazy afterwards. The authority of conventional medical opinion had determined for her what was "normal" and what was not. "Insanity" was the only name and meaning she'd been given for her experience, a meaning seared repeatedly into her bewildered skull with megavolts of electricity.

Adrift in the storm-tossed sea of her inner world, my mother had somehow found a small raft to cling to, one that her doctors agreed to call "reality." They allowed her to come home. But she was never the same. She lived bound tightly to the mast of that little raft, still floating upon that sea, never quite normal, never quite mad. A madness, held down by drugs and willful effort, lived beneath the surface.

Throughout my childhood I'd known the confusion and dread that come from living in the presence of repressed insanity, vicariously experiencing the unbearable tension of one who constantly lives "holding it all together." This potent complex of experiences was deeply ingrained in my cellular and emotional memory. I knew better than most that "they" did "bad things" to people who "weren't normal." They had taken my mother away, and returned a different, tormented creature in her place. Now a strange world had opened inside of me. And I feared it was that world that had swallowed my mother, and taken her laughter and her peace away.

One week passed after my return. Then two. The continuous jungle vision had lasted only two days. The unusual lucid state, with its disturbing energy rushes and odd perceptions, remained. I grew increasingly worried. I'd hoped my return to work and all the rituals of ordinary life would anchor me once again in my former reality. But it didn't. Then something happened that seemed to take things one step further.

For the past six months, Dean had suffered the recurring painful medical condition of a bleeding bladder. His physicians had run every test on him, yet they could neither explain nor cure his condition. One Saturday night, two weeks after my return, I saw in a dream a vivid, poly-colored neon-electric vision of an unfamiliar plant. My dream struck me as interesting but not significant.

The next day Dean and I took a Sunday afternoon hike along the coast. On our walk back, I glanced down beside the path and saw the identical plant I had seen in my dream the night before. Intrigued, I plucked it and took it with me, intending to identify it later on. On the way to our car, Dean stopped to use the restroom. When he came out, he told me, with some distress, that his bladder was bleeding again. His condition, by now somewhat routine, was by no means a casual matter. We went straight home to call the hospital and arrange to see a urologist immediately.

When we got home, Dean rested on the couch, and I went into the bedroom. I needed to briefly compose myself before calling the hospital. Still holding the little plant in my hand, I sat on the bed, closed my eyes and prayed for help and guidance. As I prayed, I spontaneously saw a clear image of a pan of red Jello setting. This odd vision was as vivid as the previous jungle visions I'd had. Then I went into the living room to call the hospital. Dean told me his bleeding had stopped. It was his last bout. The condition did not return again. A serious medical condition had been mysteriously healed.

Not long after that, I managed to identify the "dream plant" I had picked on the coast. It was horsetail, which I learned has historically been used as a folk herbal remedy both for kidney and bladder ailments, and also as an astringent to stop bleeding and stimulate wound healing. It seemed a remarkable coincidence. Yet it didn't really explain the mysterious healing. True, I had stumbled upon a traditional herbal medicine for Dean's condition after seeing it in a dream, *yet it had not been directly applied.* My pharmaceutical training most certainly had taught me that medicine, in order to have pharmacological effect, must either be ingested or applied directly to the body.

My rational side discounted the event as mere coincidence. Another part of me couldn't help wondering...had Dean's healing occurred by non-physical means? Had this herbal "medicine" been "applied" in some mysterious fashion? Fascinating as these ideas were, they also seemed potentially delusional. And I didn't want to follow them too far out on that limb. Besides, it could all be explained away. My red-Jello-vision could be disguised wishful thinking. I might have heard of the medicinal uses of horsetail years ago, and then forgotten about it. And the dream, finding the plant the next day just before Dean's bout of bleeding, and the prayer and his apparently spontaneous healing? Well, explaining it *all* away turned out to require a bit of imagination.

But it was not an isolated incident. Soon after that, a new even less rational development intruded. It started on my local nature walks, and again involved plants. One morning while strolling along a favorite pathway, I suddenly had the distinct impression that the plants were speaking to me. Tuning my attention, I found that I could make out their meanings so clearly I could almost take dictation. They seemed to be communicating to me directly, with charmingly poetic personalities. Here, for example, is some of what the tiny blue forget-me-nots said to me on April 27th, 1995, during a hike near my home in Tennessee Valley.

"My delicate nature could be passed over as just another cute little forest flower. But pay heed, for within me there exists both light and love. And as I am, so you are also. We plants are a community of beings, just as you are, and we

have specific medicines to share with you. We shine our light upon facets of you."

I was intrigued. I looked around to make sure I wasn't being observed. And before I could rear my skeptic's head to dissect the experience with my analytical scalpel, or explain it away with reason, I said a few words back to the little plant. I couldn't resist!

"What medicine?" I asked the little patch of blue flowers.

"Pay attention to what you feel when you are around us," the little flowers—or at least the voice in my head—answered back. Then they spoke no more.

"Where on Earth did that come from?" I asked myself in disbelief. And I walked away from the little talking blue flowers as quickly as I could. Imagine me, a jaded pharmacist, talking to plants!

So, where on Earth did it come from? Did the flowers really speak to me? Was it just some sweet, crazy, poetic voice in my head? The scientific truth of the matter was, and is…I haven't the slightest idea. And it didn't stop. A week or so later, while walking through the suburban neighborhood surrounding the clinic during my afternoon break at the pharmacy, I thought I heard a soft voice whisper from above.

"Up here…"

I stopped and looked up, but all I could see and hear were the fan-shaped leaves rustling on an ornamental boulevard tree. Then I felt and heard a soft rushing sound in my ears and head, like the sound of the sea in a conch shell. My mind and eyesight felt unusually clear and sharp in that moment. Looking down, I noticed the fallen leaves under the tree, and without thinking, I picked up a couple and took them with me.

That night, I looked for the leaf in an herbal reference book I'd recently bought in a health-food store. I found a sketch in the book of a similarly shaped leaf. When I placed the unusual bi-lobe, fan-shaped leaf I had found beside the sketch of the leaf in the book, they were identical. It was the medicinal leaf of the ginkgo tree. Ginkgo, the book said, increases the blood flow to the head by dilating the peripheral blood vessels. Therefore it is used to enhance mental functions. Was that the source of the rushing sensation in my head and the sudden feeling of mental clarity...increased blood flow? Ginkgo's properties are fairly well known now, but not then, and not to me, consciously at least.

I was even more intrigued, excited and worried than before. Had I felt the ginkgo's medicinal effects without ingesting it? Or was this more like mother's madness? She had been able to tell who was at the door before the doorbell rang, and she had been diagnosed a psychotic.

Still, we intuitively sense people's qualities. Why not the medicinal qualities of plants? But the whisper...had I heard it? Or imagined it? I didn't know. And the idea that I might be suffering from hallucinations or delusions still worried me.

The rational scientist in me tried not to believe or disbelieve, but to observe what happened and see if it could be proved valid or true. On one level, I found these unbelievable conversations disturbing. On another level I enjoyed them. And often, as with the ginkgo and horsetail incidents, there was a kind of "crazy logic" to the information I received. So did it come from the plants, or from some mysterious place in my own psyche? I cannot say. And I may never know.

But I'm getting ahead of myself. At that point, I had no

comfortable relationship to my new-and-not-a-bit-improved life. I wanted my old one back, no questions asked. I wasn't sure how much more of this I could take. A rational scientist and a mad mystic seemed to be fighting for possession of my mind. Personally, I was rooting for the scientist. It didn't occur to me that these two apparently opposing perspectives might blend harmoniously in a unified and complementary whole.

Ready to face the worst, I sought a professional psychological assessment. I'd get a prescription for some pharmaceutical magic bullet, if it could help me. I made an appointment with a highly recommended local psychotherapist with a reputation for helping people navigate unusual states of consciousness. I had unaccountably wandered into one, and I definitely needed a map of the territory.

I showed up on time for my appointment, afraid to tell him what I was experiencing, and afraid not to. Yet I needed help. So I poured out the whole story to him through my tears. I told him about my mother's madness, my career as a pharmacist, my trip into the rainforest, my encounter with shamans, my spontaneous jungle visions, the talking plants, and my fear for my sanity. I was reliving my childhood nightmare: *"If I tell you who I really am and what I really think and see and hear and feel, you will drug me and hurt me, you will lock me up and tie me down and fry my brain with electricity…like you did to my mother."*

He listened to me quietly for half an hour, hardly interrupting, not seeming fazed in the least. He even seemed kind and reassuring. When I had finished my outpouring, he said with calm matter-of-factness, "You are going to lead a very creative life."

What the hell does that mean, I wondered? Is that

supposed to help me?

"I just want my life back," I retorted.

"You're not crazy," he said. "You're having a spiritual emergence."

I didn't believe the first part, and the second part sounded like pie in the sky from where I was sitting. I had expected some tidy clinical diagnosis, and perhaps a prescription for Thorazine or some other "rational" medicine.

Instead he said, "We should work with this energy and this opening you've been given. Follow it more deeply. Let's see where it leads you."

Easy for you to say, I thought. And what's this "we" stuff? If this leads to the nuthouse, I'm the only one who'll be going.

Next he gave me some suggestions for dealing with the energy surges I was still experiencing. He even told me it wasn't odd for a pharmacist to have a deep spiritual connection with the plant kingdom, since most pharmaceuticals have their origins in plants. He also gave me some articles to read on shamanism which, he implied, was connected to pharmacy and to my unusual experiences. All of these things would be validated over the next two years in a most extraordinary manner.

But for now, my fears kept me in confusion. I read the articles on shamanism, but didn't find them reassuring. My mother's story, with its sadly-ever-after ending, haunted me. I could not calmly accept what was going on in me. I had ongoing sessions with the psychotherapist. I was a resistant, but utterly persistent client.

And work with the energy I did. Sometimes I'd wake up at 2:30 A.M. in full throttle, feeling like I'd drunk a quart of espresso. I'd wake up Dean and drag him with me on fast walks through the neighborhood until the energy surges subsided. The energy came in other forms, such as automatic picture drawing which I felt compelled to do at times. I'd never done art of any kind, nor do I today. But that seemed to be the outlet this super energy demanded at that time.

When the urge came, I'd grab colored pens and paper and begin, without thinking or planning. Usually within two minutes, an entire picture would be drawn automatically through my hands. The drawings were always thematically similar, overlaid with plants or flowers, often animals with flowers tattooed on their skin, or women flower spirits, or drawings of myself with plants growing out of my body. (I still have these drawings on my living room wall.)

I'd never been interested in plants before. I had only one plant in my home, an African violet. It was green, therefore I watered it. This was the extent of my botanical interest before my trip to the Amazon jungle.

Only Dean and my psychotherapist knew what I was going through. I certainly didn't tell my family or my professional colleagues. I continued work as usual in the HMO pharmacy, holding it together during the day, and letting the energies out at night in my walks and my automatic drawing. My life went on like this for many months, and to a certain extent I grew used to it. But underneath it all, I still lived with the fear that I might be going crazy.

I clung to a faint hope that this condition would run its course, like a flu or a virus, and work its way out of my system. Maybe it was neurological. Yet these unusual experiences would soon be the least of my problems. They were hints of madness, just the iceberg tip of an ordeal that would soon engulf my physical body, my marriage, and my career of over two decades. The next eighteen months of my life would lead me into a vortex of personal, physical, and professional collapse. If my dark night of the soul was a trip down a jungle river, then the boat carrying me along, steered by some faceless navigator, was headed for the falls.

CHAPTER 4

DEATH
AND REBIRTH

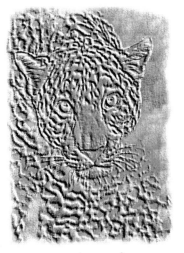

very night the same dream was repeated. A crowd of angry people searching for me. I hide in terror behind a big oak tree at the edge of a forest. They find me, grab me and drag me off, struggling, screaming, fighting for my life. Then, out come leather straps; oddly, they look like old-fashioned leather medical restraints, the kind once used to strap to a gurney patients about to receive electroshock treatment. But in the dream there is no gurney. They strap my wrists tightly behind me and lead me to a clearing where a stake rises from a pile of kindling. And they tie me to it. I'm in agony. I know I'm about to be burned at the stake for speaking my truth. But I don't know what this truth is. How can they do this, I keep asking myself? How can they do this? It is unthinkable.

They light the fire and I scream in helpless terror, consumed by the flames, consumed by my own fear. Night after night I burn in this fire. Night after night I die. I don't know why this dream keeps repeating. Was I a witch whom the Holy Inquisition burned at the stake in the Middle Ages? Am I reliving in symbolic form my mother's agony, witnessed during my childhood, rekindled in me now by my own fears for my sanity? What truth was I dying for? What deeper message did this dream convey? One interpretation didn't escape me—I as my mother bound to a gurney in a madhouse, burned with electric fire because her truths seemed crazy to others.

During this period, a slight pain developed in my wrists at work, precisely where the leather straps were tied in my dream. Was there any connection between them? As weeks passed, the pain began making it difficult to fill prescriptions. Was my pain psychosomatic, a somatization of a dream state? The more the pain in my wrists grew at work by day, the tighter they were bound by the leather straps in the dream at night. I tried to ignore it.

The nightmare with its extreme emotional distress seemed like more craziness to me. My life was difficult enough with talking flowers, whispering trees, late-night energy surges and bizarre automatic art from Meepzor, or wherever it came from, channeling through my hands. Not to mention the periodic migraines I'd suffered over the past two decades.

I desperately wanted my psyche fixed and my perceptions returned to their old track. I wanted my ordinary, respectable, middle-class life back. I wanted to be a contented pharmacist dispensing medicines that worked to patients who were healed by them. But none of these things seemed within my reach. My life was out of control. So I watched helplessly, and waited to see what would happen.

"Work with the energy," my psychotherapist said, urging me to allow the energetic process I was resisting out of fear.

"How can I? It's working *me*!" I retorted, almost writhing in my chair.

"Try some yoga," he suggested matter-of-factly.

"Isn't that some sort of cult?" I asked, squinching my face.

He must have had his private chuckles over me, a middle-aged Minnesota Catholic gal who thought yoga was a cult, catapulted into a world where plants spoke to her, visionary art spontaneously streamed out of her hands, and dreamlike hallucinations flooded unbidden into her mind. Spiritual seekers scoured the globe looking for shamans and gurus, diligently performing exotic practices, exercises, and rituals, hoping to trigger the very phenomena Miss Minnesota Connie was now trying desperately to get rid of. And all she wanted was a safe, normal, middle-class life as a local pharmacist. Yes, he had to be amused.

To my relief, neither my psychotherapist nor my husband ever suggested that my experiences or my behavior was delusional or psychotic. They were very supportive. Yet I felt on-guard around most of my professional associates, fearing they would misunderstand. I felt trapped in between two worlds—the old one I'd been raised in, and the new one I'd been catapulted into—and at home in neither. Maybe my profession, with its rigid, scientific-materialist worldview, was crazy-making to me at this crucial point in my life. Maybe I just needed to spend more time with like-minded people.

I once heard a story about a kingdom where the water was somehow poisoned. Anyone who drank it went mad. Eventually all the subjects drank the water. But not the king. Soon the whole mad kingdom believed the king alone was insane. The king knew all his subjects had gone mad, and why. But in the end he became so burdened by his isolation that he drank the water anyway, simply to join them. Not that I believed everyone else was mad. But I understood the king's sense of isolation. I wanted to be with people who understood me, who could help me get through whatever it was I was going through.

At my psychotherapist's urging, I attended a yoga class at a local community center. I stood in the back of the room, watching people fold themselves in half and turn themselves into pretzels. My body wasn't that limber. So I half-heartedly did the poses, relaxed, and let go of all expectations.

The yoga teacher's words faded away. Then my body started to shake as it had during don Francisco's healing. Energy surged through me like rocket fuel. It felt wonderful! My wrists didn't even hurt. Maybe there was something to this yoga. Maybe other people like me were having these experiences. Maybe I'd been tense all my life, suffering from spiritual repression, and this was just how it felt to have the stopper pulled out of the bottle.

Meanwhile at work, the pain in my wrists grew worse. I finally went to see one of the clinic physicians. He diagnosed it as work-related carpal tunnel syndrome, or repetitive stress disorder, and prescribed ibuprofen as an anti-inflammatory medication, and physical therapy. The phrase "repetitive stress disorder" seemed significant. It sounded like my life for the last five years, the one I had wished would change before it actually began to change. It was a relief to learn that the pain in my wrists was an actual physical problem. This allowed me to dismiss pesky thoughts and disconcerting theories about its psychic, past-life, or dream origins.

The medication dulled my physical pain, but left my psychic pain intact. And the burning-at-the-stake dreams continued. Many prescription refills and months of physical therapy later, I was in worse shape than ever. My pharmaceutical faith was at an all-time low. The pain in my wrists was becoming unbearable. I was depressed, distressed, wandering through a dark tunnel with no light at either end.

One day, while reaching for the bottle of ibuprofen on the top shelf of my medicine cabinet, I felt a lump in my throat. I looked in the mirror at the place where I felt it, but saw nothing. Then I stretched, turned my neck at an odd angle, and saw a marble-sized lump. How long had it been hiding there? Alarmed, I immediately made an appointment to see one of the clinic physicians.

A needle biopsy identified a benign growth on my thyroid gland. Because of its size, I was sent to see a surgeon. Up two floors I went, to the surgery department, my appointment card in hand.

"May I help you?" asked the registration clerk, balancing the phone on her shoulder.

"I have an appointment to see one of the surgeons," I replied nervously.

"With whom?" she asked.

"Hmm…let's see. I don't remember *which* doctor I'm supposed to see," I said, fumbling for the appointment card with the doctor's name.

"Sorry, we don't have any *witch* doctors here," she replied wittily.

"I know. I have to go all the way to the Amazon to see my witch doctor," I said, amused by my own response.

Odd how she'd picked this particular comment out of the air. And maybe I *did* need to go to the Amazon and see a witch doctor, a shaman. The subject was on my mind, and now I was hearing it from a surgeon's receptionist. The rainforest had made a profound imprint on my psyche. In spite of my fears and all that was happening to me, part of me wanted to return to the Amazon to learn the secrets of the rainforest. I wanted to learn whatever shamans like don Antonio knew. But I was in a frying pan now, and going back to the jungle would be to jump into the fire. Let's just get this lump taken care of, I told myself.

When I saw the surgeon, I wanted to know everything about my thyroid, and my body, as related to the lump. Other than his assurances that removing a lump on a thyroid was a routine procedure, he was not a fount of information. To him, the problem was an objectified physical lump and the solution was purely mechanical. A standard healthcare training perspective: Illness = problems with body parts. My problem contained no mystery. My surgery was like changing the timing belt on a car. Simple, straightforward, cut-and-dry.

I had been trained to the same perspective. Now I didn't feel that way, so this surgeon and I had no point of contact. To him, I was a mass of assembled body parts, one of which needed a piece removed. To me, I was so much more. In his detached, matter-of-fact presence, I recalled how don Antonio had looked into my eyes, so present and emotionally connected to *me*, listening attentively to my words, even, it seemed, to my soul.

And I recalled the shaman don Francisco's comments after my tobacco healing ceremony nearly a year and a half ago: "She has a block in her neck." Had he sensed something energetically, long before the physical manifestation of this lump? Was it a coincidence? Or could a native shaman, with no M.D. degree, diagnose a medical condition with no physical examination and no lab tests run? My belief system was being challenged on every level. I wished I'd paid attention to his remark at that time.

I wanted to believe the surgeon. This *was* a cut-and-dried operation, the simple removal of a tiny lump that was not me, from a much bigger lump that was. But the shaman's comments now seemed to imply something more. Maybe the lump was an effect, and the "block" was a prior cause to be addressed. If that were so, merely removing the lump might be the equivalent of merely pruning a plant potted in toxic soil. How could I get to the roots of the problem, to the heart of the matter in me? This the surgeon could not tell me. He recommended only surgery. And I arranged a date for it with the receptionist before leaving his office.

But I had a gnawing feeling and I went to get a second opinion, from another Western-trained surgeon. Maybe I should have asked a shaman. I felt a rapport with the second surgeon, who listened carefully to my concerns. I felt comfortable enough to tell him what the shaman had said about a block in my neck.

"Well, that's how he sees it," he said. "It's as good a diagnosis as any."

I liked his openness. But he also had no clue as to prior causes. All we really knew was that there was a lump in my neck, a fact any surgeon, shaman or five year old child could verify. The rest, East or West it seemed, was theory. We agreed that he would do the surgery several months hence. No hurry, as it was a benign growth and my thyroid functions were fine.

So I went back to work. I was bound to the pharmacy by golden handcuffs. More accurately, I clung desperately to a highly respected, well-paying career with which I was completely disillusioned. I kept trying various medications for the pain in my wrists. None of them did the trick. I increasingly identified with my many complaining, unhappy, despairing customers whose medications, provided by me, also didn't work.

Finally the severity of the pain in my wrists forced me to quit my job. I was now unemployed and without a profession. I knew I'd never work in a pharmacy again. But I still had to make an income. I didn't know what to do. So much was happening all at once—disability, surgery, the loss of my career and possibly my mind. But sadder losses were to come. In the midst of all this, Dean and I realized that our marriage of nearly twenty years was over. We were both devastated. He was going through his own changes, and he now moved on to a new location and started a new career. I hunkered down to lick my wounds, worry about my sanity, and prepare for my upcoming lumpectomy surgery.

The surgery brought one more surprise. After the operation, the surgeon told me that the lump on my thyroid was malignant—cancer. They would have to remove my thyroid. Misfortune comes in flocks; when it rains, it pours; the wheel of the gods grinds slow; and in my case, they also sent tornadoes.

Eighteen months had passed since my visit to the Amazon. I had no job, no prospects, no marriage, no peace of mind, and no faith of any kind. Everything I wanted had been taken away. And the one thing I had—cancer—I wanted to get rid of. I was spiraling on the edge of a vortex of death...physical, emotional, and spiritual. Three days after the first surgery, I went under the knife again. My thyroid was history.

I sat alone in my house for weeks, recuperating, with nothing before my face but the darkness of my life. During that period, Marin County experienced its worst storms in fifty years. One night the storm was so fierce it knocked all the electricity out. It kept on storming, and it took a week to get the power back on. More tornadoes from the gods?

I ate cold food and washed with cold water the surgical scar that marked the cancer. Only candles lit the darkness of the night. The storm raged on with howling winds and torrential rains. Then the floods came, turning streets into rivers, invading houses, burying cars, and sweeping them off roads into ditches.

I felt a bit like Job, but I couldn't take it personally. And my house and car, on a hill and out of danger, were spared. But the access roads below were flooded, and I was cut off from the outside world. Cold and alone, my food supply dwindling in the fridge, my spirits and my immune system in a tailspin, my fear for my sanity reverted to plain old fear of death. My God, I began to think, I really could die! In retrospect, it may have been a healthy perspective shift.

One night, as the storm raged outside, I had the nightmare again. The angry crowd bound leather straps about my wrists, tied me to the stake, and lit the fire. But as the flames licked my flesh for the hundredth time, I didn't feel the burning. An unknown force lifted me out of my body. I was no longer a terrified, bewildered victim inwardly wailing "Why?" This new self called out to my tormentors, "You can burn my body, but you can't burn my spirit!" As I stood in the spirit of truth, in my own name, the leather straps binding my wrists fell away and I stepped down from the burning stake into the crowd. I felt no hatred for them. I forgave them all. In that moment, I knew freedom. When I awoke, the storm outside had subsided, and I felt a deep inner calm.

Weeks went by and the inner calm remained. At least I never wandered too far from it to find my way back. I seemed to be recovering on every level—physically, mentally, emotionally. Gone the fears of madness and dying. Yet something in me had died, or was dying a necessary death...my old belief systems, my resistance to my own inner changes, my fear of the unknown. My prolonged ordeal, and the cancer, with its spectral taste of death, had shifted something deep in me.

Out of work, I spent more time walking and talking with the plants. Crazy or not, I enjoyed these private "conversations." To balance spirit with science, I enrolled in some local classes on herbalism, eager to learn the chemical constituents of medicinal herbs. I felt the most sane in nature, among plants. And whatever made me feel good, I decided, was the medicine I needed. My psychotherapist agreed.

On my way to the first class in an outdoor medicinal herb garden, I felt one of my migraines coming on. Rather than go home to lie down, I decided that being outdoors in the peace of nature might help. Our instructor had us sit beside the herb garden while he delivered his introductory remarks. I sat in the summer grass leaning back against an old oak tree, in its welcoming shade. A country breeze swept through my hair, caressing my throbbing temples. Barely hearing the instructor's words through the pain, I closed my eyes and tried to relax. Then, faintly, I heard a soft voice next to me.

"Eat me," it said.

I opened my eyes and looked over…no one was there. I closed my eyes, and moments later the tiny voice beckoned again, *"Eat me."*

I snapped my eyes open and searched around. My gaze settled intuitively on a little green plant in the herb garden beside me, waving its leaves in the afternoon breeze as if to catch my attention. I felt like Alice in Herbal-land—more at ease than ever with the experience of talking plants. I no longer wasted my mind arguing with myself over whether plants could talk or not. I accepted the messages that came as something to be taken seriously. As long as they weren't telling me to rob banks or blow up national monuments, I saw no reason to fret.

Well, I thought, if this little plant wants me to eat it, why not be a gracious garden guest? But I did want to check first with the instructor. I got his attention and asked him the name and medicinal uses of the little green plant.

"That's feverfew," he said. "One or two fresh leaves chewed daily, or taken in capsules or tincture, can relieve or prevent migraine headaches."

Need I have asked?! I picked two leaves of this friendly little plant and chewed them on the spot. I also obtained a seedling from the gardener to plant at home, and later purchased some feverfew capsules from a local health-food store. It did the trick. Two weeks of continuous use mitigated intractable migraines I'd suffered for the past twenty years.

This was more than surprising. Over the years I had tried every migraine preventative, curative, pain pill, and anti-inflammatory medication known to modern pharmacy…to no avail. In despair, I had finally given up medicating my migraines, believing I'd just have to live with them. Nature had once more proven her superior pharmaceutical skills.

My hero! I called feverfew "the little leaf that cured the big headache."

This herbal cure fueled my passionate interest in learning the healing properties of medicinal plants. Not that feverfew works the same for everyone...no remedy does. But it further convinced me that medicinal herbs can fill a significant gap in modern medicine's treatment of a wide variety of ailments. After several months of intensive study, I apprenticed to a wonderful "alternative" physician.

Dr. Dee, as she liked to be called, a sprightly young woman with golden-white hair, was one of those courageous pioneers who had been exploring natural medicine for decades. She treated her patients primarily with herbs, supplementing her practice with conventional medical remedies, recommending modern pharmaceuticals and surgery only when necessary.

Dr. Dee and I worked out a mutually beneficial arrangement...she would teach me how to treat a variety of ailments with herbal remedies, and how to make these remedies, in exchange for my assistance in her herbal pharmacy. We worked together out of a big old house, its bedrooms converted into exam rooms. While she treated patients, I worked in the former kitchen, now an herbal pharmacy. It was suffused with the pungent, earthy smells of an old-fashioned pharmacy. I cut the leaves, flowers, and roots of various medicinal plants taken straight from the garden, then put them into jars of alcohol to steep. Weeks later, the alcohol had extracted the active ingredients from the herbs, turning them into medicinal tinctures. I also cooked up delicious, honey-based herbal cough syrups on the stove-top that soothed and satisfied raspy throats, and mixed heady, aromatic essential oil-of-lavender with golden yellow calendula to make an all-natural, first-aid cream. I felt I had stepped into one of the historical pictures that hung on the walls in the Minneapolis College of Pharmacy.

This was the pharmacy I had imagined as a young girl, infinitely richer than the sterile count-and-pour assembly line where I'd spent the past two decades. I had stepped into a timeless past where pharmacy merged with mythology…I was an ancient alchemist in her laboratory, concocting life-prolonging elixirs, a fairy tale witch brewing mysterious potions in her bubbling pot. I was apprentice to Hippocrates, preparing herbal remedies for his patients in ancient Greece. Ironically, if this Father of Medicine came back to practice today, he'd be called a quack no matter how many patients he cured!

I watched many of Dr. Dee's patients recover using herbal remedies, and the conventional medicines and procedures she prescribed when appropriate. Her integrated approach to healing taught me much. She used both in appropriate measure, and didn't throw out the baby with bathwater. I was amazed by the public's response to her practice. Dr. Dee was booked-up a year and a half in advance for new patients. And her patients were extremely loyal. They liked her "try nature first" brand of medicine, which often worked. She was also a healer *inside*. She cared deeply about her patients, and they felt this.

I'll give a few case examples that I witnessed. Mr. Koch, a thirty-five year old salesman, had suffered recurrent sinus and upper respiratory infections for three years running. He'd been on routine prescription antibiotics, but he wanted to get off of them. His job required almost continual airline travel, and it seemed that frequent prolonged breathing of stale, infectious airplane oxygen, combined with a stress-depressed immune system, might be at the root of his problem. We sent him home with some echinacea to take three times daily. Two weeks later, his infection had cleared up completely. After that, he continued to take the echinacea just before, during, and immediately after his flights. This echinacea got him off antibiotics, and healed his sinus infections.

Ms. Albright, a forty-two year old career woman, came to us with chronic stomach problems and a case of gastrointestinal reflux. She'd been self-treating with various over-the-counter antacids for the past six years. (Antibiotics and antacids are two of the top-selling medications in the United States. No wonder our pharmaceutical and medical industries are doing their best to subvert the growing interest in herbal remedies!) Ms. Albright jokingly claimed to own stock in Glaxo, the manufacturers of Tagamet, a stomach acid-reducing drug which she consumed like candy. But she wondered if all these medications might in fact be disturbing her digestive tract. So she came to Dr. Dee looking for a natural alternative.

An initial consultation revealed that her problem had even more complicating factors. Ms. Albright also routinely took aspirin and ibuprofen for her "workaholic headaches." Both medications are known to irritate the stomach lining. So, she was in fact taking antacids to counteract the side-effects of the anti-inflammatory medications taken to relieve headaches caused by stress resulting from overwork and lack of rest…you get the picture. Her stomach problems were an all-too-common example of a pharmaceutically-induced condition.

A conventional doctor may have indeed written Ms. Albright a prescription for yet another drug to add to her medical daisy chain. As a conventional pharmacist, I would have mechanically filled this prescription and sent her back to her life as it was. The root causes of her condition would not have been addressed. Years down the line she might have ended up like millions of elderly people out there, suffering a variety of pharmaceutically-induced symptoms. She would have a medicine chest full of counter-active, counter-productive, unnecessary prescriptions, the daily combination of which would produce nothing resembling a state of health.

Instead of the above route, we had her stop taking all of her medications. (And folks, *don't* try this at home without the supervision of an experienced herbal doctor!) I whipped up some marshmallow glycerite to soothe and protect her stomach. Dr. Dee prescribed a cup of chamomile tea five times a day to soothe and heal her gastrointestinal tract. Chamomile tea, a mild relaxant, besides the calming ritual of tea-sipping itself helped her to relax and release stress which reduced her headaches. Six weeks later, Ms. Albright happily reported back to us that the only "drug" her shopping cart contained these days was her chamomile tea.

As for me, I was far happier concocting and dispensing herbal remedies in this converted house-clinic than I'd ever been filling prescriptions as a conventional pharmacist. Apprenticing with a Western M.D. in the use of natural herbal medicines showed me this plant-based medicine was not just an "indigenous thing." (Herbalism was indigenous in every part of the world before the advent of modern pharmacy.) I saw firsthand how receptive people are to natural alternatives to conventional medicine. I witnessed firsthand the true healing power of many natural plant-remedies. And I gained a healthier respect for, and a growing interest in, the medicinal wisdom of "indigenous" herbal healers everywhere, from

American physician herbalist Dr. Dee, to Peruvian rainforest shaman don Antonio.

One day, while brainstorming/worrying on the compelling topic "how the hell am I going to make a living," I had an idea. Why not form a professional association to educate practicing pharmacists in the use of medicinal herbs? I knew other pharmacists could benefit from the education and experience I had received in this area. And this would give me an opportunity to pass on what I had learned, while deepening my own knowledge in the field.

I now strongly believed that herbalism, a growing counterculture movement for the past thirty years in the United States, was destined to enter mainstream medicine. It was an idea whose time was coming. And I hoped to help usher this idea into practice. I believed that people, if properly educated, would see the wisdom of integrating natural and pharmaceutical medicines. They would also feel it in their bodies, not to mention their pocket books. In many cases, prescription medications are far more toxic and expensive than their natural counterparts. Why not give nature's remedies a chance, in appropriate cases, before prescribing chemical drugs with side-effects, for instance, where chemical means are prohibitive for any reason, or have already proven unsuccessful?

The healing properties of many medicinal herbs have long been backed by solid scientific research. Yet most pharmacists and health care professionals were still largely oblivious to, or skeptical of, their medicinal properties and potential. I knew many other pharmacists out there who would be interested in learning what I had discovered.

So the Association of Natural Medicine Pharmacists (ANMP) was born. It was just a name given to an idea at first. Yet once I took this step, I began to wonder how open my fellow pharmacists would actually be to the concept of natural medicines. Still, I scraped fifty dollars out of my dwindling savings and had some brochures made at a local copy shop. I handed them out at professional meetings, and sent them out to mailing lists of pharmacists I had bought. If the response was good, I'd invest more in professional graphics and educational materials.

Within a month, the pharmaceutical community and media had caught wind of the ANMP's formation. The idea of a pharmaceutical organization devoted to the study of herbal medicine struck a chord of interest, particularly in the pharmaceutical journals. Whether they saw merit in the idea, or simply saw it as a curious or controversial topic for magazine stories, my phone started ringing. I began giving interviews. Articles about ANMP soon began to appear in professional pharmacy journals. Soon I discovered a small but growing group of pharmacists opening to the idea of natural medicines. (Now, after nearly a decade in existence, I am proud to say that ANMP has educated tens of thousands of pharmacists throughout the United States on natural medicines and is still going strong.)

The plant world that had figured prominently in my crisis over the past two years had now given me a new career. With one foot in the world of Western pharmacy, and another in the world of traditional plant medicine, I now began educating my first-world peers on the benefits of a second world in which I was still a humble apprentice. The explosive energies that had plagued my body and tested my sanity for the past two years were now yoked to my new career. I was cancer free, single, and making a living on the cutting edge of my profession. Most importantly, I was free of a deep-rooted fear, carried since childhood, that I was doomed to repeat my mother's tragic life. And I felt anything but crazy now as I moved steadily along my own path. I felt reborn, inspired, and full of gratitude.

The more my connection to plant-medicine deepened, the more I felt the rainforest calling me to return. In a dream I saw shaman don Antonio uttering the words he had spoken to me in our conversation in the rainforest: "You have enough energy to be a shaman yourself." For me he was the embodiment of a plant-medicine healer. I wanted to see him again. I wasn't exactly sure why, or what I would do if I found him. I didn't know if I would be able to find him. And to try meant that I would have to return to Peru alone.

I wasn't quite ready to fly to Peru and wander into the Amazon jungle. But I had a feeling I might do so in the not too distant future. For now, I simply prayed to be guided on my path. Whatever was meant to be, so be it.

CHAPTER 5

JUNGLE MEDICINE

Alone, I stepped onto the dock from the *rapido,* the speed boat I'd been lucky enough to find in Iquitos. The three-hour journey north down the Amazon and onto the Yanayacu tributary to this jungle village would have taken eight hours by colectivo.

My God, I thought...here I am! This was my second trip into the heart of the primal rainforest. It was as beautiful and mysterious as I recalled. But I was different, sobered and changed by a two-year ordeal catalyzed in part by events during my previous trip here.

Now here I was again, come halfway around the world seeking the hair of the dog that bit me.

Two days ago I stood in San Francisco International Airport amidst thousands of tourists in Western dress, surrounded by vast tracts of modern suburbs. Now I stood, a lone woman on a rickety wooden dock amidst Amazon locals—dockworkers unloading supplies and loading jungle produce, the camp crew, a few boatmen—separated by custom, skin-color, language barrier and worldview, and surrounded by a vast jungle seething with an unimaginable variety of plant and animal life.

A month ago I'd tracked down news of don Antonio, who was helping to plant an ethnobotanical garden in this village on the Yanayacu River where he had been born. Learning that he needed volunteers, I jumped at the opportunity to come soak up the splendor of the rainforest and learn more about its medicinal plants by tending his garden. Not too far in the back of my mind was the idea becoming don Antonio's shamana apprentice.

Nearly two years had passed since I'd first met, and last seen, don Antonio. Since then my life, and my mind, had been turned upside down and inside out. The jungle had been working its medicine on me all this time. Now, feet firmly on the ground and feeling like a different person than the naïve gringa *turista* I'd been two years ago, I'd returned to find out what don Antonio had meant when he'd told me, "You have enough energy to be a shaman yourself."

I was here to explore both the offer, if such it was, and the man who'd made it.

I unfolded my purple cotton kerchief and looked for a

dry corner to wipe from my face and neck the rivulets of salty sweat broiled out of me by the equatorial sun. Get used to it, I told myself. This is how it's going to be for the next three weeks. Ironically, I'd caught laryngitis and a cold before leaving California. A cold in the heat of the Amazon jungle? My raspy, congested voice seemed like a joke here.

I noticed swarms of yellow and blue butterflies scouring the river embankments, licking the salt and mineral traces the receding waters had left behind. They even clung to me, their probiscus tongues licking the salt from my sweat-stained T-shirt. I had now officially entered the Amazon food chain as mosquito prey and substrate butterfly lunch.

"Cone-ee! Hola! Cone-ee, aqui!" a familiar voice shouted my name in a thick accent. I recognized don Antonio's voice, and two of the few words of Spanish that I knew. I sharpened my focus, sorting through the small crowd of barechested dock-hands glistening with sweat, bearing cargoes of ripe *plátanos*, the jungle bananas, and heavy water jugs on their bare shoulders. Then I saw him. He had a light blue bandana wrapped around his forehead.

"*Hola!*" I called enthusiastically, my voice squeaky as a beginner's violin.

It felt good to see don Antonio's face again. He navigated through the dockhands with the ease of a river snake moving through open water and we soon stood face to face. There was a brief, awkward moment on both sides…what was the protocol for brown and white, male and female, South American teacher and North American student? But if we listen, the heart speaks clearer than words and determines its own protocol.

"*Muchos abrazos,*" don Antonio smiled disarmingly (I later learned this meant "many hugs"), and we exchanged a warm hug. I felt I'd been welcomed by the magnificent rainforest itself.

Don Antonio's assistant, Manuel, helper in his medicinal garden and our translator, now stepped forward and introduced himself. He was younger than don Antonio, and smaller in stature and build, with a sincere face and a broad smile. I felt good knowing he would help to bridge the language barrier between me and don Antonio. Chatting eagerly, we three walked along the docks, with Manuel translating and adding his own asides. Don Antonio noticed my croaking voice, which sounded like one of the ceaselessly chattering river frogs.

"*Resfriado*, Connie?" he asked, which Manuel translated as 'Got a cold?' I told him I did. "*No hay problema*," he said. "I'll take care of it as soon as we get to the gardens."

I imagined fresh ginger from his garden made into a soothing tea for my cold. I wondered how much I could learn in three weeks about Amazon medicinal plants. Who knew, the "materia medica" in his garden might hold secrets that could change the course of medicine as we know it.

As we walked, Manuel told me this medicinal garden project was close to don Antonio's heart, since it was so close to the village of his childhood. He said even before don Antonio started this garden project, he had come here periodically to teach the villagers about medicinal plants, to work as a healer, and to visit old friends and family members.

Finally we arrived at the camp, situated along the river a fifteen-minute hike from the village. Its hub was a large octagonal *maloca,* or communal house, a simple platform with a palm-leaf thatched roof and screens all around, raised on stilts to accommodate unpredictable seasonal changes in the river water table. When the glaciers of the high Andes melted, the Amazon and its innumerable tributaries rose, often flooding the surrounding jungles. Right now, in low-tide season, the river was fifty yards from our camp. But Manuel told me that in the full-river season, the camp usually bordered the river's bank.

I could hardly wait to enclose myself in the protective screens of the maloca. Word of my arrival seemed to be spreading among the jungle mosquitoes who had already honed in on me. My nordic Minnesota bloodstock was surely a rare delicacy in these parts. Don Antonio pointed out my sleeping quarters off one end of the maloca.

"After you've unpacked, have lunch and a siesta," he told me, "Manuel will bring you to the garden. It is not too far into the jungle."

I went up the wooden steps and entered my quarters through the screen door. Inside was a wooden bed and mattress covered neatly with a mosquito net. A pitcher of water and a wash basin sat on a small table in the corner. I almost never nap, but all the excitement and the intense humidity had made me lethargic. The jungle heat precipitates a natural slowing down of all organismic life. Sooner or later, every living thing subsides into a jungle rhythm. And I found myself sinking into the peace of jungle time...no time...*mañana* time. I lay down on my cot and quickly drifted into sweet sleep.

I dozed for a couple of hours, unconsciously sensing changes in the temperature and angle of the sun. I woke to Manuel's voice outside my room.

"*Vámonos*...time to go to the garden."

"I'm coming," I said, voice still raspy and congested.

I got up, feeling refreshed, and went out into a soothing late-afternoon breeze. I was just in time to see wee Manuel disappear into a thick, twelve-story emerald forest whose multi-layered cloud-high canopy hid the sky. I ran down the maloca steps and followed him in.

On entering the jungle path I discovered that the breeze was restricted to the open spaces of the camp. This primal jungle, the rainforest equivalent of old growth forest, was a sauna...hot, wet, and claustrophobic, conducive to lethargy, sweating, rotting and dying, but not to breathing. Its ambience combined an unbelievably dense mixture of smells—pungent, sweet, rank, earthy—floating in an almost Jello-like humidity...smells of river water and fetid swamp, chlorophyll, blooming orchids, ripe melons, rotting vegetation, mildew, rain, sweat, and death. The primal smells of nature herself in all of her stages, from conception through birth, death, disintegration, and reincorporation back into the elements. This is the jungle theater, nature endlessly giving birth, and ultimately devouring all that she has created.

Add to that an equally dense thicket of sound—fluttering, creaking, whimpering, shrieking, whispering, buzzing, croaking, hooting, crying—a zoo gone manic, a cacophony of bird, insect, animal, and vegetable life. Add to that again the enchanting other-worldly avalanche of exotic vegetation such as the mysterious stilt trees each with dozens of stick-like legs but no solid trunks, corkscrew woody vines, zigzag monkey ladder vines, and ropy lianas, all hung in a tangle with a thousand plant-lets whose varied leaves were camouflaged and indistinguishable—except for the elephant leaves that were larger than myself. It was all teaching me just how insignificant, small, and alone I was.

I hurriedly caught up with Manuel and followed him closely. If he even got ten feet ahead, any curve in the path made it seem as if he'd been swallowed up, and I felt lost. I also felt like a potential jungle snack. Any large predator might be hiding in any thicket, invisible to my untrained eyes. The jungle works on one's imagination. At one point I began to hear the forest whispering my name ever so softly… *"Connie,"* over my shoulder, behind my back. The first time it startled me.

"What?" I called to Manuel.

"I said nothing," he replied. "We'll be there soon."

I knew it must be the leaves rustling. But it happened several times, leaving me with an eerie feeling. Jungle paranoia, I decided.

When we arrived, don Antonio was waiting for us outside his *tambo*, a small, open-sided thatched palm hut built on a raised platform at the garden's edge. The garden itself was around five sparsely planted acres, so far containing around 50 varieties of medicinal plants. My job would be helping don Antonio plant another hundred varieties. He invited me in, and Manuel went over to talk to two local villagers casually working at the far end of the garden. Once inside, don Antonio motioned for me to sit on a handmade wooden bench. I sat down facing a hammock strung up at the other end of the hut. Don Antonio looked at me in an odd way. I felt that he was seeing more of me than my physical body.

Without a word, he lit a cigarette—not an ordinary cigarette, but a shaman's cigarette, a full 4 inches long and a half-inch in diameter, hand-rolled from a very strong local *tabaco* known as *mapacho*. He took a *shacapa*, a leaf bouquet, in his other hand and started to shake it over me like a maraca, gently tapping my head and moving down body with a rhythmic tempo. As he did so, he began to murmur and chant a strange, high-pitched, atonal song called an *ícaro* that went from nasal twang to falsetto. It took awhile for my ears to get used to this ícaro which seemed nonsensical compared to Western music. "Ney ney nai ney," he sang, tapping the shacapa all over my body, taking breaths and puffs of smoke between phrases, and blowing tobacco smoke all over me...whoooosh...pff...pfft...mostly over my head and chest.

After five minutes of this unusual ritual, I noticed how pleasantly relaxed and energized I felt. There was something haunting, mesmerizing about these healing ícaro. Their primal sounds merged with the gentle rhythmic flopping of the shacapa leaves on my body, and went into my soul somehow. It felt strangely soothing.

A few minutes later, don Antonio finished and motioned for me to go lie down in the hammock. When I did, he put his index finger in front of his pursed lips, signaling me to quiet down. Then he gently brushed the shacapa-mussed hair from my eyes, patted my head, and left the hut. Within moments, my breathing relaxed, my tight chest opened and my congested nose and head cleared, just as he had promised at the dock.

At the same time I felt like I was swooning in a force or energy that made my body tremble, as it had during my encounter with the shaman don Francisco on my previous visit. Excited and a little frightened, I called out don Antonio's name. There was no violin rasp, no froglike croak. My voice was back.

This healing defied all of my rational, Western medical assumptions. Not even my experience in the herbal clinic had prepared me for this. Healing via pure ritual...not even a cup of ginger tea! My response was equally irrational; I found the incident very upsetting. I was glad my cold and laryngitis, against which herbal remedies and decongestants had proven futile, were gone. But I expected a cure to have some solid basis and a plausible explanation. But I had none. I had come to learn about healing beyond Western pharmaceuticals. But I wasn't prepared for so much "beyond" so soon. Was this mysterious medicine magic, or placebo?

"It's almost dinnertime," Manuel announced a few minutes later, poking his nose discretely into the tambo.

Manuel, noticing I was a bit shaky, assisted me as we walked back to the camp. All the way I grappled with this healing conundrum. I reviewed my "case" and groped for rational explanations. In our Western allopathic medicine, you treat conditions with their opposites; that's what "allo" means, "opposite." For congestion you take a counter-medication, a de-congestant, whose pharmacologically active ingredients change your physiology and cause the congestion to subside. But here I was given nothing that remotely qualified as a medication, or any other kind of counter-actant. Instead, I was sung to, blown on with tobacco smoke (which should have aggravated, not alleviated my congestion), and bonked on the head and chest with a bouquet of leaves by a man who'd never attended school, and had no formal degree of any kind. I felt silly, confused, and out of my league. Admit it, I told myself, you were cured by a witch doctor!

Don Antonio was not far behind us on the walk back to camp. In his hand he was carrying a bunch of green *hierba luisa*, lemon grass, freshly picked from his medicinal garden. At camp, don Antonio proceeded to fold the long, grassy stalks into pieces that fit neatly into a tea cup. As he poured hot water over the grass-filled cup, the fragrant lemony scent of the medicinal herb permeated the humid air.

"Here, drink this," he said. "It's soothing for your throat and your mind."

I took a sip of the aromatic tea, I then spoke up. "Don Antonio, how did you get rid of my cold so easily? And without any medications," I prompted Manuel to translate. Inquisitive by nature, don Antonio asked the questions first, "Can I learn to prescribe your modern medicines? Can I go to school in your country and become a physician in a hospital? How do the doctors in your country treat colds and other illnesses?" Don Antonio must have read my thoughts about the differences in medical approaches.

I explained to don Antonio how basically a Western-trained physician uses various laboratory tests, X-rays, and CAT-scans to "see" inside patients and make a diagnosis. A prescription is written based on the results of those tests. Don Antonio was staring at the ground, listening thoughtfully. He looked up at me, shook his head and responded, "Well then, I am not interested in learning your medicine. I don't need any machines in order make a direct diagnosis. I can see into my patients with my own eyes. And my medicine is medicine from nature and spirit, which heals not only their bodies but their hearts and souls, too. I'm sorry but I'm not interested, because *your medicine does not have any magic in it*."

I didn't have anything to say. My mind was racing with questions. Had his "magic" cured my cold? Was this some sort of "invisible medicine" of the spirit? Were his senses somehow so heightened that he could actually "see" inside people?

I was subdued during dinner, noticing a sharpening of my own senses. Fresh fish, boiled in rainwater, and mashed bananas never tasted so good. Don Antonio observed me, but said nothing. We ate in silence. After dinner, I went to bed, exhausted, and fell quickly asleep.

I awoke the next morning, completely refreshed and invigorated. My dilemma of the previous evening had evaporated.

"Hey gringa!" said Manuel cheerily as soon as we finished breakfast, "You'll want to work in the garden in the morning while it's cool." Cool? It was already 90 degrees in the shade! "Bring lots of water with you," he added knowingly. "And don Antonio says to wear your rubber boots, and bring your raingear and a towel."

With an average of 210 inches of rain a year here, and an average temperature in the high 80's to 90's, no wonder the average humidity was only slightly less than a heated swimming pool. How long would a towel stay dry? Ten minutes? Wasn't a towel here a rainforest version of the proverbial snowflake in hell? Should I bring a towel to dry the towel? Of course I withheld my wry comments, and brought a towel.

The tools of a rainforest garden are simple...a shovel, a wheelbarrow, a machete, and a broom. No rake. My first assignment was a Sisyphusian task...sweeping the garden floor clear of the leaves that fall in a continual rain in this kingdom of plants. I felt like I was sweeping waves on the shore back out to sea. I knew who would win.

I also noticed Manuel's habit of bolting at the sight of anything that looked like work. He knew what needed to be done, and how to do it. But he preferred to show me how, and then leave me to it. Not that I minded. I had volunteered to come. I didn't dare ask don Antonio if I could be his apprentice. I decided I'd just work diligently in his garden for the next three weeks and see what happened.

So I worked in silence, sweeping the earth, my mind, buzzing from my breakfast coffee, full of a thousand questions I could not ask don Antonio because Manuel, our translator, had disappeared. Around mid-morning, I noticed don Antonio picking limes from a garden tree. He cut several in half and squeezed their juice into a glass of water. I kept sweeping, and salivating. It was oppressively hot. Out of the corner of my eye, I saw him blow tobacco smoke from one of his mapacho cigarettes over the limewater. Then he brought it over to me and motioned for me to drink it, saying, "*Es refresco.*" "Refreshing" I understood. I gratefully gulped down the tangy liquid and returned to my sweeping.

As I continued to work, I noticed my state distinctly shifting. I became more aware of my surroundings. I seemed to see more clearly. I felt a new depth of feeling, of connectedness to my surroundings. I noticed that everything really was alive, literally. To notice this was to be absorbed in life. Nature was truly a "sensurround" event.

I continued sweeping the leaves of the towering cecropia trees, and the fallen fronds from the tops of the trunkless, otherworldly stilt palms. I lost my sense of time and merged with the timeless jungle. I swept the maroonish pod-fruits of the achiote tree, the fallen leaves and lavender flowers of the regal *jacaranda* tree. I felt nature alive, pulsing all around, and me not separate from it. I was a creature doing my part in creation, sweeping leaves in the jungle. I found myself weeping uncontrollably, supporting my heaving body on the broom handle, overwhelmed by a profound sense of connection with the Earth, of awe at the sacredness of nature.

Had don Antonio done something to the water? Was this an effect of prolonged exertion in these potent surroundings, or of a combination of random factors that could never be traced? I was embarrassed by my tears. Get a hold of yourself, Connie, I told myself. You're a trained healthcare professional. You're here to learn about medicinal plants and native healing practices, not to cry over swept leaves. Get a hold of yourself. Just keep on sweeping.

Around 5 P.M., don Antonio returned from the far corner of the garden with Manuel in tow. I'd been sweeping now for six or seven hours with occasional breaks. Don Antonio grabbed his washbasin, motioned for me to follow him. One-by-one, he collected portions of five different plants— *murcura, ajo sacha, hierba luisa, clavo huasca, and guayusa.* Then he went around to the back of his hut and put them into a basin of rainwater he'd been saving. He showed me how to manually crush these wonderfully aromatic plants in the water until it formed a vibrant green soup. Manuel explained that don Antonio was making a healing herbal bath called a *limpia,* which means "to cleanse."

"You are about to receive a healing with this limpia," he added. "It is an important ritual in the rainforest shamanic tradition. Now follow the shaman to the creek with your towel."

Don Antonio led us out of the garden, through the jungle and down to a shallow creek. Then he motioned to me to remove my clothes. "*Calma, calma,* (relax)" he said in his most reassuring voice. The idea of taking my clothes off in the jungle with two indigenous men I barely knew was a bit unsettling. Manuel left, perhaps sensing my reluctance. But I was more curious than fearful, and I hadn't come all this way to let my Minnesota Catholic prudery interfere with a shamanic initiation.

I shed my clothes and don Antonio motioned for me to stand in the creek. In silence, he began to pour the green aromatic plant bath over my head and down my body. It was certainly refreshing. He continued pouring the limpia over my head.

Watching the play of shadows and late afternoon light on the creek, I sensed a presence, or was it only my heart opening, my body melting away as the last bit of limpia trickled over me. Was this ecstasy, or was I only present at last? How many times my rational mind would ponder variations of this question. Was my "altered state" only a natural state experienced by someone cut off from nature and armored from simple feeling? Are we so cut off from life as it is, that to be simply, fully present is ecstasy, an epiphany? Is the healing power in nature, and the trick of shamans, that they bring us into natural states of consciousness that only *seem* altered compared to the repressed states in which we spend most of our lives?

Don Antonio looked knowingly at me, and nodded in approval. After I dressed, he motioned for me to follow him, and we returned to the garden and sat down on the bench outside the hut. Eager for information, peeking out from under the towel as I dried my hair, I asked Manuel to translate for us.

"Don Antonio, what is the purpose of this herbal bathing ritual?" I asked.

"This limpia is a sacred healing that washes away negative energy and restores *energia positiva*, positive energy," he answered through Manuel.

"Could you give me the list of plants that you used?" I asked.

I was thinking "Western pharmaceutical" again; if I used

the same plants and performed the same actions with others, imitating what don Antonio had done with me, I could give people the same healing. Don Antonio thoughtfully rinsed out his washbasin, and with it the flies that had collected in the bottom.

"I pick different plants to be used," he said, "depending on the energy of the patient and what I want to accomplish." (Only later did he give me the list of plants he had used on me.) Head bent, focusing on the task at hand, he looked at me sharply out of the corner of his eye from under his brow and added, "For this healing to be powerful, you must do it with great respect. Unless you have a spiritual relationship with the plants you use, it doesn't work."

"What was in that lime drink you gave me earlier?" I asked next. "Nothing but a good dose of spirit and lime," he answered with a chuckle. "You wanted to learn about the garden and my healing work, didn't you? Then you must experience the Earth and its plants with your heart, not just with your mind. That's the difference in our medicines. My medicine has magic in it, yours does not. Spirit does the healing, not science. Science is good, it is knowledge. But spirit has the real power."

The idea that I had a lot to learn was sinking in. I had naïvely believed that studying shamanism, if don Antonio were willing to teach me, would be relatively straightforward: memorizing information, learning about plants, performing rituals...sort of like college. I was smart, disciplined, and had much pharmaceutical knowledge. This, plus my passion for herbs, I thought, would make me a quick study as far as shamanism went. I'd pay attention, ask intelligent questions, memorize the answers, and quickly master the art of healing with medicinal plants. Right?

Au contraire, Connie, was the feeling I was now getting. I was steeped in the Western assumption that the healing was in the medicine, the pill, the mechanical process, the material elements of the cure. Don Antonio was turning me to another dimension of healing. The shaman, according to him, healed through his spiritual relationship with plants, nature, spirit, and the patient. This was a completely different paradigm of healing than the one I had learned in college.

I blurted out several more "intelligent" questions in rapid fire, which don Antonio patiently answered. Then he concluded bluntly.

"With all respect, you don't know what you're talking about," he said, his voice full of kindness. "I'm sorry, it is not possible to explain to you in words the world of the spirits and how I work with them. It is a different world than this one we are accustomed to seeing."

Then he rose to leave. He had nothing more to say.

It was shortly after sunset. I lay under my mosquito netting mulling over the day's activities, thoughts swarming like a cloud of mosquitoes in my brain. Picking up my flashlight, pen, and journal, I wrote, "December 20, 1996." Where to begin? How to make sense of what had happened to me these past two days? The question that kept coming to me was, "Where am I?" Yet it wasn't about a location on a map, but a location in my mind. My reality compass was scrambled.

It had started when don Antonio healed my laryngitis. Then, his explanation of healing physical ailments with spirit defied all my medical training. And the profound altered states, absurdly triggered by nonsensical rituals, hadn't helped. Don Antonio blowing smoke at me, singing bizarre songs, tapping me with leaves, giving me lime water with smoke blown over it, and pouring herb water over my head while I stood naked in a creek.

Yet I had been opened somehow to the sacredness of nature, to a deep love and respect for the Earth and its plants that I had never experienced before. This I couldn't dismiss as some theatrical trick a shaman was playing on a gringa. Deep down I knew I had experienced a healing and a teaching of life-changing importance.

However simple and apparently "uneducated" don Antonio seemed, his undeniable personal authority and medicinal wisdom inspired trust and respect. His words made sense; they felt profound and true. Intuitively, I knew he was right. Without a deep spiritual connection to nature and its medicinal plants, I could not become a true shamanic healer. Don Antonio clearly had an intimate relationship with the plants he used as medicines. But what was I to think when he talked about the world of spirits? Despite my experiences in the United States with horsetail, ginkgo, and feverfew, I didn't believe in the spirit world the way he seemed to, and this was a significant difference between us. Was this why his healing seemed to have magic?

A river of medicines had passed through my hands in my 30 years as a pharmacist, yet I had no spiritual connection with the medicines I dispensed, nor with any spiritual powers or beings. Nor did any of the doctors that I knew. This "spiritual" component or vision that defined shamanism was precisely what Western medicine lacked. We put all our eggs in one basket. Our medical institutions were antiseptic yet impersonal. We had powerful drugs and sophisticated technology, yet we lacked the spiritual foundation and insights that could produce truly wise and potent healers. We avoided intimate relationships with our patients (not to mention our medicines), and failed to acknowledge the spiritual mystery of the healing process. And if spirit healed, as don Antonio said, then conventional medicine was significantly crippled by its failure to address these issues.

Don Antonio clearly embodied the essential qualities of a healer that I felt were absent in my own tradition. They were what I had come here to learn. My education, I now saw, was no mere college course in jungle pharmaceuticals. It entailed a paradigm shift about the nature of healing, even the nature of reality. It required acceptance of a seemingly irrational dimension of life, and a relinquishing of a limiting rationality indoctrinated into me by my upbringing and my scientific training.

From where I was now, this seemed a risky and very worthwhile proposition—a continuation of a journey I had been on for the past two years, that had tested me, and made me stronger. And I was willing to continue being put to the test, if that was the price of the knowledge I sought. I had come on a quest to learn the nature of healing beyond pharmaceuticals and Western paradigm medicine. Now, after 24 hours with don Antonio, I felt more certain than ever that I, too, wished to become a shaman, whatever that meant.

I worked hard, sweeping and clearing the garden over the next several days when it wasn't raining. I was taking to the jungle. I learned to wield a two-foot machete, which I swung back and forth close to the ground, weed-whacker style, to remove unwanted newly sprouting plants. I donned my Indiana Jones hat, slung over my back, whenever it started to drizzle. My rubber Wellies kept my feet dry, and

protected my ankles and legs from snakebites and my
machete.

By the time I swept and weed-whacked my way across
the garden, which took several days, the area I'd cleared the
first day was already overgrown. You can't keep the jungle
down. Manuel, for whom even paid work was undesirable,
thought I was crazy for volunteering to do this. We had two
different work ethics: mine Protestant, his mañana.

But even in my rubber boots, my feet were never really
dry. Thanks to the humidity, they generated micro-climates
all their own; each contained its own sweltering tropical zone.
Not surprisingly, after a week's work, my left big toe contracted some sort of "jungle rot," and began throbbing to the
beat of an unknown microbe. I looked at it one morning as I
was getting ready for breakfast before work. It had worsened
severely overnight. It was now quite swollen and painful, and
the nail had begun to float and ooze a nasty fluid. I couldn't
even get my boot on.

I reached for my first-aid kit for some antibiotic cream.
Being a pharmacist, I had of course brought a more-than-
adequate first-aid kit along. Then I paused. Why not see what
jungle medicine the shaman prescribed? Wasn't this what
I'd come to learn? So I put on my rubber flip-flops and went
in search of Manuel, and some breakfast. After downing our
breakfast and morning coffee, we headed down the trail to
the gardens through dense jungle canopy speckled with
morning sunlight. We arrived to find don Antonio sitting on
the bench outside his hut, sharpening his machete on a
whetstone.

"Don Antonio," I called, catching his attention. He
looked up and I pointed to my left foot. *"Problema!"* I
shouted in my gringa Spanish.

I hobbled over and the shaman got up from his bench to make room for his patient. He squatted and examined my reddened toe, pushing and prodding at the toenail. Then he spoke, and Manuel translated.

"Your toenail may turn black and fall off. It's not serious yet. But I don't want it to turn into a blood infection. It could go up your leg and into your groin area. Then what would I do?"

Don Antonio half-comically threw up his hands. But I knew it was potentially serious. As the only source of local healthcare, don Antonio took his shaman's role seriously. If complications set in, we were at least three hours by high-speed boat from the nearest medical facilities. I didn't tell him I had powerful antibiotics in my first-aid kit. I wanted to see how well his jungle medicine worked on its own.

"Let's gather some plants and make an herbal foot bath for you," don Antonio said. "If the inflammation doesn't subside within a few days, we may have to slice open your toenail with my machete. But we'll see." I wasn't sure if he was joking. But I was definitely rooting for the herbal footbath over the machete pedicure.

I hobbled through the garden behind don Antonio while he gathered leaves from seven plants from his outdoor pharmacy. They were *casho, piñón blanco, paico, and sangre de grado* (used, he said, to treat infections); *papaya macho, and camote* (useful in treating fungus); and *arnica* (used both as an antiseptic and an anti-inflammatory). Next he methodically tore them into little green shreds, dropped them into a basin of water and added ordinary table salt to the concoction. The salt I understood, the rest I simply trusted. I felt like the ancient pharmacists who grew and harvested the plants, brewed the mixtures, and compounded the final medicines. It was worth hobbling around the jungle garden in pain to live a moment of original pharmacy.

Several times a day over the next two days, we would gather more of these fresh plants and brew another batch of foot-soak medicine. What most struck me about the treatments was the unquantifiable ingredient in don Antonio's ministrations, the care and attention he showed to me, his patient. I'd never felt this level of sensitivity and intimate concern in a Western medical setting, not even in the throes of my bout with cancer. I saw how this level of compassionate attention implied in the medical term "attending physician," was a largely unfulfilled promise in the West.

"It's ready, Connie," don Antonio informed me through Manuel. He gently put my left foot into the herbal bath, the fourth one on the second day, and carefully worked the green medicine under the toenail as best he could. It occurred to me that I hadn't been so cared for since I was a baby. He reached for a towel and began to dry his hands.

"Just let it soak for awhile," he said.

I sat with my foot in the basin, staring out over the garden. Don Antonio stepped away to chat with Margarita, the camp cook, passing by at the end of her long workday. I saw by their gestures and glances my way that don Antonio was discussing my case with her. A moment later, she came over and asked me, through Manuel, how I was doing.

"*Bien*, just fine," I replied. "I'm in good hands." She nodded supportively.

Now José, the camp night watchman, came through the gardens from the other direction. He too joined us to ask how I was feeling, and spoke a few heartfelt words of encouragement. Then the three of them chatted in Spanish with each other for a few moments. The same thing had happened yesterday. I was struck by the genuine concern for my welfare on the part of the locals who knew me.

It dawned on me how, in a tribal society, the health of each member was of great importance, as each one contributed something of essential value. An unwell mother couldn't cook for her family. Injury to a hunter could mean insufficient meat for the group. If the shaman were incapacitated, there was no tribal doctor to deal with medical emergencies. And so on.

Back home, when I was ill or injured, I took a pill, applied some kind of medication, put on a bandage and went back to work. And no one much cared one way or the other. Feeling this group care and support made me realize what a deprivation its absence in modern culture truly is. I recalled how painfully isolated I'd felt for two years while going through my own health crises. This human "care," largely missing in modern healthcare, is perhaps the most important medicine any of us, including our doctors, can give, and the essential healing prescription no pharmacy can fill.

In the fading afternoon, don Antonio and I sat alone on the bench outside his hut at the edge of the garden. Margarita, José, and Manuel had gone. I pulled my left foot out of the footbath and reached for my towel, but don Antonio shook his head. "*No,*" he said, and he put both of my feet into the plant bath. *Both feet,* my skeptical mind reacted? *Doesn't he know anatomy,* my superior pharmacist self observed critically? *Only my left toe's infected, not both my feet.* Maybe this was primitive medicine after all.

It was the second full day of this treatment, and my toe showed no improvement, though it also wasn't getting any worse. Still, my skepticism increased as he began pouring the green plant bath all the way up both legs to my knees. Due to the language barrier, I couldn't ask his rationale for this unusual treatment.

Next, out came the shaman's cigarette. Don Antonio lit up and began puffing on the strong mapacho tobacco, blowing clouds of smoke about my legs. No songs this time, just tobacco smoke blown with great deliberation. A few minutes later, the smoke-treatment done, don Antonio dried my legs with a towel.

"*Cena*, (dinner)," he said matter-of-factly, and motioned toward the camp. Nothing more was said.

That night, I had unusually vivid dreams. I saw kaleidoscopes of bright swirling colors and surreal dreamscapes. At one point I found myself sitting alone in a bare room on a wooden chair. A shadowy figure appeared in the doorway and came threateningly toward me. Though terrified, I stood up on the strength of my own two feet, faced the figure, and held my ground. In the dream, this was all it took to defeat the frightful apparition. The dream then "popped" and I slept calmly for the remainder of the night.

The next morning before breakfast, while taking a shower, I leaned over to clean off the pus that accumulated on my infected toe each night. There was no pus. The redness and inflammation had also subsided. The only thing left to heal was the raw-pink new skin around and just under the toenail. I was surprised, considering its grungy appearance yesterday, and its seeming lack of progress. It had practically healed overnight.

I dried, dressed, and found Manuel, and we went straight

to the shaman's garden. I wanted to show don Antonio my healed toe, and I wanted Manuel there to translate. We found him on the bench outside his hut, surveying his garden.

"*Mira*! Look, my toe is healed," I exclaimed, walking up to him with no trace of a limp. He nodded knowingly and examined the toe. "How did it happen so quickly?" I asked.

"We weren't getting good results with the plant baths, so I decided to do a shaman's healing on you," don Antonio said, with Manuel translating. "I invoked the spirits with tobacco to give you strength in your legs to fight off this infection."

I recalled last night's dream, and how I had stood my ground, both feet firmly planted, to defend myself against the apparition. Now the image made sense. I told don Antonio my dream.

"You had a weakness in your legs," he responded, shaking a stern finger at me. "That's why the microbes were able to attack you there. Germs are everywhere, constantly bombarding us. We have a natural ability to ward them off," he continued. "But where we are weak, we are vulnerable to their attacks. Your dream showed you the spirits working in your body. The shaman calls upon the spirits to give you strength to defend yourself, and the energy to heal."

"Don Antonio," I began, "you've given me several healings since I've been here…first my cold, then the limpia, and now my foot. Sometimes you use herbs and sometimes you use your shaman's methods. How do you decide which to use?"

"I usually first give my patients certain plants to eat or drink," he replied. "It's important to have a lot of *vegetal*, a lot of green plants, in your blood. This fortifies you beyond the healing ceremony. If the plants aren't working, or if we need to speed up the healing, or if it's clearly only a spiritual problem, then I go straight to the spirits for help."

I paused to absorb what he'd just said. Having experienced firsthand the efficacy of his healing powers, I couldn't help but be intrigued by this explanation. Yet it was still hard to accept the idea that my physical foot needed a spiritual healing, or the help of invisible spirits, in order to fight off living microbes, or that a physical infection might have spiritual causes. What exactly was spirit, and how did it heal physical maladies? If spirit was an intelligent life-force that animates the body, perhaps it could physically recharge the body's energy, maybe even boost the immune system, which would help it to fight invading microbes. But could a healer activate spirit and direct it in this way? Don Antonio not only seemed to think so but also even seemed able to do so.

There were other conundrums. If don Antonio indeed invoked spirit, or spirits in his healing practice, where did they come from? The plants themselves? Was spirit literally in the tobacco, or in the limpia? Did it come from the shaman, from the mysterious ethers, or any other far-fetched place? And was spirit more important than the pharmacologically active ingredient in the plant?

I was genuinely baffled. Western medicine is founded on the presumption that physical maladies have physical causes, not spiritual ones. A malady with emotional roots we often label "psychosomatic" (read "imaginary illness"). Mysterious healings with no apparent material basis for their cures we often attribute to "placebo effect" (read "imaginary cure") or call "spontaneous" (read "how the heck did that happen?"). These "medical" terms give the false impression that we understand phenomena that are inexplicable. We name a mystery and mistake it for knowledge.

Suppose, to explain my toe cure, I label the infection "psychosomatic," and say don Antonio's herbs and rituals are "placebos" which have triggered a "spontaneous" cure. What has been explained? *The source of my healing remains mysterious.* And in the light of my own experience, *all* such explanations now seemed like Western voodoo, explaining nothing. To continue believing such non-explanations, I now saw, closed my mind to genuine mysteries, and to the possibilities they contained. Clinging to rigid belief-systems that could not be proven seemed a kind of lobotomy. And I saw now that the reason I had long performed this operation on myself was to deny my own ignorance, and to shield myself against life's humbling mysteries.

But maybe it was better to be humbled, and accept my ignorance. Maybe I needed to simplify my mind, by opening it. Maybe the answers I sought were staring me in the face, embodied in this simple shaman. Spirit heals, don Antonio had said, and spirit is everywhere—in the shaman, the patient, and all of nature. To learn his kind of medicine, it seemed I needed to stay open to mystery, to possibility.

I could feel myself moving closer to asking don Antonio to take me on as his apprentice. The clarity was coming. But I didn't quite have the courage yet.

"Don Antonio, how do you know if a physical problem needs a spiritual healing?" I asked. "And does the spirit that heals come from you, the plants, or somewhere else?"

"It's all the same," he answered softly. "In the end it cannot be explained."

His simplicity penetrated my complicated thinking. There was no magic formula, no answer to "cure" the mystery. The shaman understood without knowing the answers, and healed without knowing ultimately how he healed. This was the "irrational" element at the heart of all healing. I gazed out over this native medicinal garden, feeling the depth of this mystery. I knew I would need time to digest don Antonio's words.

With my foot mended, I returned to my garden work with full vigor, making myself useful and asking lots of questions. I cleaned and tended the garden beds and got to know the names and medicinal uses of all the plants. "*Qué es esta?*" "What's this?" I asked don Antonio many times a day about each plant I encountered. I also practiced using the Spanish phrases I'd acquired from ever-present Manuel, who preferred interpreting to gardening.

"*Es Santa Maria,*" don Antonio tickled the long, fingery, fruit-like stalks and heart-shaped leaves of one plant. "I make tea of its leaves for people who feel sadness in the stomach." He then picked a large six-inch leaf, rolled it up, and placed it across his forehead. "It's also good to use like this for headaches."

"And this one, don Antonio?" I asked.

"*Esta es piñón rojo,*" he said. "Its dried fruits are a laxative." Then he added, "It also helps to keep out bad spirits. I use its big red leaves for those who are spirit-possessed."

My insatiable curiosity, which kept me pointing and asking, was matched by don Antonio's infinite patience, and his seemingly inexhaustible plant knowledge. Some plants, he said, were used for physical ailments, others for emotional or spiritual problems, and some, like the Santa Maria and piñón rojo, healed at all levels.

Late one afternoon, near the end of my three weeks of volunteer work, don Antonio asked me and Manuel to come to the garden at 8 P.M. for a special healing. At 8 P.M. in the jungle it is pitch-black night, and there is no night darker in my experience. So, after a shower and dinner, at the appointed hour, I was walking through the jungle with Manuel behind me, and don Antonio ahead holding a kerosene lamp.

Halfway to the garden we entered an enchanted Fantasia realm…the sky beneath the black backdrop of the jungle canopy 20 feet above suddenly became a dizzying firmament. Thousands of fireflies soared, blinking surreally like Christmas lights. I felt my heartbeat fall into syncopation with their rhythmic, hypnotic flight.

The jungle comes alive at night, and my ears rang with the profusion of nocturnal animal cries. I heard the indescribable, enchanting pebbles-dropping-in-water "ploop" calls of the dusky-green oropendola birds; the deep-throated "beeps" and "warps" of the never-silent toads and tree frogs; and the prolific, ever-changing cries of the inventive douroucouli—the noisy night monkey—lent a primal richness to the evening's symphony. I even heard an elusive jaguar in the distance announcing his nightly hunt with a 300-pound growl that chilled the hot night air. This sound brought home the stark reality that in the jungle there is no certain survival, no respite from death, only an endless hunger, punctuated by the nightly terror of prey; day or night, it's eat or be eaten.

Don Antonio, holding his lantern out before him, seemed a spectral shadow leading us into the endless green foliage. As we entered the open garden clearing by the hut, I looked up and saw the fire-works multitude of stars twinkling in the equator sky. Don Antonio set the lantern down and quietly motioned for me to sit on the wooden bench. Then he got out his shaman's tools—his shacapa and his tobacco—and began. He worked on me for an hour and a half straight, puffing clouds of tobacco over me, singing his haunting, magical ícaros, shaking and tapping his shacapa rhythmically on my body.

My mind wandered through the usual assortment of thoughts from the day's events. After an hour, when he was still working with me, I began to appreciate the intense effort he was clearly exerting on my behalf. This demonstration made me aware that healing is partly due to the literal offering, or sacrifice of life energy the healer bestows on his patients. Being the recipient of this energy and attention did make me feel good. And I found myself basking in this soothing energy.

Then a voice deep inside me said, "That's not enough. This isn't just about you. It's time for you to sacrifice something of yourself, and give to others." What does that mean, I wondered? As a pharmacist, I had always been once removed from the sick, safe behind a counter, separated from patients by a literal barrier. Now the voice within me said, "If you want to be a healer, you cannot hide. Look deep within, face what you fear, give yourself away, and be willing to bear the responsibility for helping others."

As don Antonio finished the healing, I noticed how hot I'd become. It was an internal heat, different from the heat of the jungle. I stared at the light of his kerosene lamp, its glow at least five feet in diameter. I blinked and looked up into the firmament of fireflies that seemed to merge into stars beyond. All was glowing.

Don Antonio took a sip of water and asked me how I felt. I told him about the internal heat and the energy glow. And then I told him what I'd understood, that the time had come to face my fears, that I was willing to give myself up and take the responsibility for becoming a healer in order to help others as he did. My chest ached and I felt naked speaking my truth, as if a war was being fought in my heart. I felt how long I had closed my heart and held back from the spirit world because of my fear of insanity. But that fear had somehow melted during this healing. The unwilling in me had become willing. My heart was open.

Don Antonio gave an approving nod and patted me on the shoulder.

"I want to apprentice with you, don Antonio," I continued blurting words. "I want to become a shamana and learn the secrets of your medicine."

"I can see that," he said gently. "I respect your Western medicine, just as you respect my shaman's medicine. Yes. I will take you on as my *alumna*, my student." Then he looked me in the eye, and with great seriousness, added, "Much *disciplina* will be required on your part. It is not an easy path. You will be tested many times. If you are willing to follow my every direction, I can teach you. The rest will be up to spirit."

I nodded, agreeing with my eyes. Then he bid us a good night's sleep and went into his hut for the night. Manuel took the kerosene lamp, and I followed him along the jungle trail back to camp. But despite my heartfelt conviction about this path that I was choosing, part of me couldn't help wondering on the way back, "What have I gotten myself into?"

CHAPTER 6

APPRENTICESHIP TO THE VINE OF THE DEAD

L et's look at you."

Don Antonio held me at arms length to get a full view... always the first thing he does upon my arrival from the United States.

"Have you been following the disciplina, the shaman's discipline?" he asked shaking his finger at me, ever the tough taskmaster.

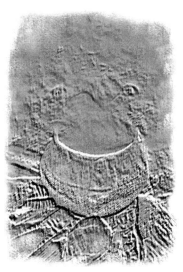

A year had passed since don Antonio had formally accepted me as his apprentice. Over the year back home, I immersed myself in Spanish lessons and struggled to keep on my path as an apprentice. I considered my first meeting with him three years ago the beginning of my informal apprenticeship, and the two-year ordeal that followed as my initiatory preparation. From the start of my formal apprenticeship a year ago he had put me through a series of spontaneous "tests" which I cannot mention, as they involved vows of secrecy, and imposed on-going *dietas,* dietary restrictions—no salt, sugar, grease, or alcohol. Then, during my last visit with him six months ago, he'd upped the ante by adding a new disciplina...no sex of any kind for at least two years...maybe as many as five, he added.

As I was single and had no romantic prospects on the horizon, this hadn't seemed difficult. Just more of not doing what I'd already not been doing, only now calling it a "disciplina." But after six months of official chastity, a new boyfriend arrived on the scene, and at this first test, I fell quickly, though briefly off the wagon.

I rationalized my brief sexual interlude as an apprenticeship recess that had nothing to do with a lapse of integrity. Why, I had kept the dietas and disciplinas...except for those times I had sex...during recess. And, having broken my word to don Antonio by breaking the disciplina, now, when he asked if I'd kept my disciplina, I answered with another little fib.

"Yes, I have."

Except for those times I had sex, said a faint little voice in the back of my mind.

"Very well, then," don Antonio responded, not blinking an eye. "Let's get to work. It's time to prepare for a limpia." The purifying and respiriting limpia herbal bath at the river's edge signified the washing away of my hectic Western persona, and my entry into the spirit realms with don Antonio. I always welcomed the shift in consciousness these limpias brought—a heightened awareness, my senses more attuned to nature and my own inner landscape, and a world become more tangibly alive than the one which I normally seemed to inhabit.

After the limpia, I had a simple dinner of chicken, rice, and beans. Then, exhausted from my journey, I went to my usual room of the stilt-raised maloca and quickly fell asleep. The rainforest was coming to feel like my second home.

A few hours into a deep sleep, an otherworldly whooshing sound, like a flapping of gigantic wings in my room, startled me awake. The entity, if that it was, sounded as big as a man. With a gasp of fear I lurched upright in bed, heart pounding. I saw nothing in the room. In America I would quickly assume that I'd had a nightmare. But this was the Amazon jungle, home of the jaguar and other predators. I sat in the dark wondering…was it a dream, or had some gargantuan nocturnal jungle creature paid me a visit? Or, was it possible that something had paid a visit from the spirit realm? The events of the past three years had expanded my old assumptions about reality to include a dimension where anything was possible.

Several minutes passed and the sound did not come again. Finally I lay back in bed and went to sleep. Around midnight I woke suddenly again with a feeling of alarm. Feeling a strong urge to vomit, I scrambled out of my mosquito netting and my room and down the maloca steps in time to purge myself at the edge of the camp. Every fifteen minutes for the next hour, I was either vomiting into the jungle or relieving a case of diarrhea in the latrine. It didn't feel like any food poisoning I'd ever experienced. And it stopped as quickly as it started. I suddenly felt fine again, though a little tired, and went back to sleep.

After this tortuous night, I woke to the sound of don Antonio's approaching footsteps. Each morning during my stays, like clockwork, he would come to inquire about my dreams. Early on in our work together he had said to me, "Dreams are an important part of our lives. Some are as important a piece of news as a birth or a death."

This morning when he asked about my dreams, I told him about being awakened by the flapping wings—I was still a bit shaken by it—and asked if it qualified as a dream or something else. I struggled in my kindergarten Spanish to explain the experience, gesticulating high in the air with my arms to indicate the size of the noisy entity. Don Antonio watched my performance attentively, and then said, matter-of-factly, "That was just me...checking in on you."

"But I couldn't see you," I said. "What was that noise?"

"It wasn't me physically," he said. "My spirit flew to you. That was the noise you heard."

He was trying hard to swallow his knowing smile, and I wondered for a moment if he was teasing me. But I could see that he meant what he said. He was simply amused by my wide-eyed enthusiasm over my "big fish" story. Especially since he was the fish I was describing.

"Anything else?" he asked. "How are you this morning?"

"No more dreams that I remember," I answered. "But I did have a bout of vomiting and diarrhea during the night."

His expression grew very sober and he looked in my eyes. "You have *not* been following the disciplina, as you said you had." He was very stern. "Shamanism *no es broma* (is no joke), Connie. The limpia is a powerful ritual designed to purify. And that it always does. You had many layers of impurity. That's why you got sick. You didn't follow the disciplina, and then you didn't tell me the truth about it. I saw it in your energy field when you got off the boat yesterday." He shook his head and wagged his finger at me. "*No sexo!* That is a spiritual order!"

I felt suddenly humbled and humiliated by my lack of integrity, and my foolishness. Had I really believed I could fool the shaman *and* the spirit world and get away with it? Or that I could escape the effects of my own behavior? I had to remind myself that I had apprenticed to the spirit realm, the ultimate teacher for which the shaman is only a visible agent. I was speechless. I had no defense.

"You chose this path, Connie," don Antonio said. "I didn't force you. If you do not follow the required *disciplinas* there will be painful spiritual consequences. I must tell you this for your own good."

There was no anger in his voice. Don Antonio spoke like a caring uncle, forced by my misbehavior to admonish me, which he did without flinching. It was still a hard truth to take, and in the moment, I didn't take it too well.

"Two years of no sex of any kind? I'll die!" I exclaimed, more than half-seriously.

"That's up to you," he said. "Many ask to apprentice with me, but no one yet has become a shaman. Years of apprenticeship alone do not make a shaman. Most fail because they do not obey the rules and live the *disciplinas*. Weak commitment does not survive the testing." Then he added in his best mentoring voice, "The deeper the commitment, the stronger the medicine."

I was choking on the strong medicine of don Antonio's words. We had met the hard part that comes in any real relationship. When the bloom is off the rose, the real work begins, beyond the safety zone of superficial social protocols and defensive barriers. I felt off-balance, caught off-guard. Had

I expected the work of transformation to occur within my comfort zone, without my being painfully stripped of a few self-protective illusions? Did I expect to become a shamana, a healer, without paying the full price? Part of me had to have known it would be like this. But like most fools, I had rushed in wearing blinders.

I knew that what don Antonio offered was not to be missed at any price. He was a beacon who had helped to guide me through my dark fears of inherited insanity, into the unknown, into a spiritual dimension of life that was beneficent and healing, and yet not to be trifled with. Now he was making clear to me that to follow the path of a healer, to open to deeper states of consciousness, I had to carry my own spiritual weight by living the required disciplinas, not seek to avoid them like an irresponsible child.

Medical students enter residency and Buddhist monks and Catholic priests retire into forests or monasteries to live disciplines that make their commitment real and bring them to new levels of mastery. Now it was my turn to get real and live the disciplines of rainforest shamanism, whether I was here, or back in the world.

One of the primary levels of mastery that sexual abstinence brings is the ability to withstand large amounts of energy that otherwise might ordinarily kill you. There are such large doses of energy contained in the shaman's Medicine...best described with a capital "M"...known as *ayahuasca*.

"The name of this plant medicine, ayahuasca, means the vine of the dead."

Don Antonio settled into teaching mode as we prepared

to build the fire. Beside us lay a couple of kilos of brown twisted vines, cut in sections, with six other small bunches of plants. We had gathered them all early that morning from the jungle. For the next twelve hours we would be making the sacred hallucinogenic brew, ayahuasca, used for centuries by rainforest shamans for healing and divination. This Medicine don Antonio called his teacher, and he was in some mysterious way its apprentice.

We stood in back of his small, open-walled shaman's hut hidden in the depths of the jungle. This was the ritual place where don Antonio treated patients, made his medicines and communed with the spirit world in his work. And this was the place where we took the Medicine together, a potent part of his shamanic practice, and of my apprenticeship.

Don Antonio and I had shared these night rituals in the past, drinking ayahuasca together with his patients. The effects of the Medicine, as he often called it, produced ecstatic states of consciousness in an enchanted ordeal that is hard to describe. Besides, each experience is always different. Tonight, for the first time, don Antonio and I would be drinking the Medicine alone. My job in today's preparations would be to stir the pot and fetch water from the river not far away when the pot boiled down too far.

The shamanic medicinal use of ayahuasca seemed paradoxical to me, for both patient *and* healer took the Medicine together. It was a mutual journey into another world, a spiritual dimension, where both the illness and the cure had their roots; where a true diagnosis could be made, and effective healing accomplished.

Both Western medicine and jungle shamanism use medicinal plants to heal. But the jungle shaman accesses and harnesses the spiritual energies of medicinal plants, not merely their pharmaceutical properties. Jungle shamans perceive an energetic continuum to plants that includes their pharmacological properties, their spiritual qualities, and even their associated spiritual entities.

We humans recognize our extraordinary spiritual members—Jesus, Mohammed, Buddha, and so forth—and we flock to them for guidance and respiriting. In the same way, shamans recognize the extraordinary spiritual potency of certain plants, which they regard as teachers, or sources of spiritual and healing power. Such plants, like ayahuasca, are living spirits in the heart of many shamanic traditions.

"This Medicine will bring you face to face with your death," don Antonio had told me on my last visit six months ago, just before my first encounter with ayahuasca. "If you live through the experience, you will be privy to many secrets of the jungle that only ayahuasca can reveal."

It had been a chilling introduction meant to sober me, and to warn me of the very real risks. Ayahuasca, more than anything in my experience, is *not* to be taken lightly.

Don Antonio now slid his *cushma*, a black shroud-like ritual poncho over his head and began the sacred ritual of preparing the Medicine. The stack of brown vines and the six other plants combined to form the signature recipe for don Antonio's ayahuasca brew. Every ayahuasca shaman, or *ayahuasquero*, brews the Medicine with slightly different plant recipes, under the guidance of the ayahuasca spirit. Each passes their recipe on only to tried-and-true apprentices, who may later adapt the recipe under the guidance of the vine. All these varied brews are simply called "ayahuasca," for the vine is their common central ingredient.

The ayahuasca vines take a good twelve hours to fully release their medicine into the brew. "Have patience and respect for the Medicine-making process," was don Antonio's pharmaceutical admonition. "Strong Medicine requires persistent effort and commitment."

Don Antonio reached for his ritual mapacho cigarettes and shacapa leaf rattle, and motioned for me to bring the six additional plant medicines closer to the fire. The vine, still needing further preparation, I left alone. Then he nodded, indicating that I should drop the plants into the large clay pot filled with water that was heating over the fire. After I did this, he lit a cigarette and began blowing smoke over the vines and over the plants I was now busy stirring into the pot with a stick. He began singing ícaros, blowing smoke and rattling his shacapa over the brewing Medicine and the stack of vines, which would be added later to the brew. When he was finished, he motioned for us to sit on the two logs near the fire.

"You have been invited to walk again through the doors of initiation," he began with great solemnity, "to partake of this powerful spirit and teacher, to be healed and to become a healer."

There was a great dignity in his words, and a deep reverence in his voice for the spirit of the ayahuasca vine. This spirit, perhaps inseparable from the hallucinogenic chemical component in the vine itself, was at the heart of his shamanic religion. Now he grabbed a chunk of the brown, twisted, rope-like vine-of-the-dead from the pile to make it ready for the pot. He lay it on a stump and began beating it with a smaller log until the vine became soft and pliable. He put it in the pot with the other plants, reached for the next section of vine, and repeated the process. At one point, he grabbed the stirring stick I held in the pot and put his other hand on my shoulder.

"We're not only rendering the Medicine in the pot," he said. "We're rendering you as well. You will eventually *become* the Medicine...*if* you live the disciplina."

"Ahhh. So *being* the Medicine is how you can heal people without giving them a dose of ayahuasca or other herbs?" I asked.

"Follow the discipline, become the Medicine, and find out for yourself!" he shot back. "To become a shaman, the blindfold that blocks your perception of reality must be removed," he continued. "But no book can teach you this. No words can make you a shaman. Only the vine can do that. But be careful, *cuidado!* Always. With ayahuasca, as you know, you will walk a fine line between sanity and madness, life and death. The vine will test you many times. It is possible that you may die...*finito*," he said firmly. "So be sure of your decision to continue on this path."

He fell silent. It was quite a disclaimer...far from the encouraging, reassuring words I always hoped for. I could feel the rivulets of sweat running down my neck. Was it the heat, or the terror? Minutes passed in silence. Don Antonio was giving me time to consider, and reconsider. Then he continued speaking.

"A jungle shaman fears three things," he said. "The anaconda. The jaguar. And ayahuasca."

Don Antonio had often warned me about *el serpiente*, and *el tigre*, terrors of the rainforest, the most feared jungle predators in water and on land. He depicted them in vivid, terrifying imagery, as jungle demons with almost supernatural powers. Alligators, equally fearsome in their own right, had been over-hunted in don Antonio's territory and so were not the threat they had been in his youth.

"The anaconda and the jaguar are so powerful," don

Antonio continued, "that one man alone is defenseless against them. Both el tigre and el serpiente hunt in the night. El tigre is the most beautiful creature, and the deadliest of hunters. He is at home on the earth, in the trees, in the rivers. He climbs almost with the ease of a monkey, and swims almost like a watersnake. He is the invisible predator, the silent stalker, the swiftest striker. He leaps from behind to crush your skull and break your neck in his powerful jaws.

"El serpiente hides in the foliage near the rivers, or hangs in the trees overhead to drop down on you when you come to drink. He can swim like an eel underwater without stirring the surface. When he grabs you, he wraps you in his coils, crushes you till you suffocate and turn to mash, and then swallows you whole headfirst."

He described how they swallowed their prey in a series of muscular, ratchet-like gulps, afterward retreating to some dark jungle thicket to lie in a stupor, often for weeks, its belly slowly digesting the unfortunate creature. Don Antonio told me he had seen *anaconda grande* nearly forty feet in length weighing several hundred pounds.

Don Antonio's descriptions of the jaguar and anaconda reminded me of the dragon lore of ancient Europe. Yet these jungle creatures, their exploits and their powers were not myths, but living realities. But then life in any major city was also a confrontation with various powers where injury or death could come swiftly and unexpectedly. Maybe all humans made the same uneasy peace with lurking death, no matter what form it takes.

Don Antonio methodically pounded the twisted, serpentine ayahuasca vine and dropped the mash into the kettle hung over the slow-burning fire. Then he looked up from his arduous work.

"Anaconda grande still live in these parts, deep in the jungle," he said. "So does el tigre. Yet the shaman fears ayahuasca as he fears the jaguar and the anaconda."

His piercing glance as he made this last statement again, and the sight of him wearing that black poncho-shroud, were sobering. He had heightened the fear I was already feeling about approaching the ayahuasca ceremony. This, I sensed, was his intention…he wanted my decision to continue on this path to be made in the presence of fear and in the awareness of death.

I looked away from don Antonio's gaze into the dense jungle where anything could hide, and anything could happen, where at any moment I might become just one more helpless creature snatched to a grisly death. I felt suddenly vulnerable, adrift in a realm of powers, powers of the animal kingdom, and other powers more mysterious. In taking the Medicine I was knocking on the door of these powers. And the door would be opened. This I knew from previous experience. But previous experience did not ease my fears of what might come. I was about to enter once more the deepest jungle mystery by invoking the spirits of the vine-of-the-dead. And who knew what troubles—and perhaps wonders—I might be stirring up. This thought now filled me with an almost unbearable terror.

"So even though I have drunk the Medicine in the past, it is still dangerous?" I asked don Antonio apprehensively. My mouth was very dry and I took a swig from my canteen.

"Every time is new. It depends on how much power you have. Ayahuasca can teach you, give you visions, make you crazy, or kill you," he spoke matter-of-factly. "So you must approach it with respect. You must enter its domain and approach its spirits slowly. I determine who drinks the ayahuasca, and when they are to drink it. I must prepare them first, and that takes time…weeks, months, even years. And I give it to them only if they are clean and of good heart. First I test you. Then ayahuasca will test you."

Don Antonio held up a section of the brown, twisted vine; it looked alive in his hands. Then he lay it on the stump.

"I did not give you the Medicine during your first healings because you were not yet ready," he said. "Then you were ready and I let you drink the Medicine. But there is always a risk. So it is important that I remind you. One should not enter the spirit realms of ayahuasca alone. You need a powerful shaman to guide and to protect you. Ayahuasca is very powerful Medicine. It's not for everyone."

A loud smack punctuated this remark as he smashed his log down on the vine. The golden glow of warm spiritual feelings, the ecstatic highs, were now a pale memory. What am I doing here, I thought? A middle-aged white woman in the middle of the jungle putting her life and soul in the hands of this shaman and his spirits? Was my thinking I could become a shamana one more sign of my craziness? Yet I could not find it in myself to get up and walk away. I also knew I needed to find a deeper courage and strength in me if I were to continue.

Don Antonio fell silent again and continued pounding the fibrous vines into pulpy shreds which he put into the simmering pot with the other medicinal plants. I simmered quietly in my dilemma. Twenty minutes passed without a word between us. I stared into the shaman's brew as if an answer might bubble up, stirring the mixture with a stick from time to time. Tonight, in the depths of the jungle, don Antonio and I would drink the Medicine together. My hope was that, with his guidance, and the help of the Medicine, an answer might bubble up in me.

Don Antonio lit another mapacho cigarette, took a long drag, and blew billowing puffs of smoke over the simmering brew. After this ritual blessing gesture, he spoke a prayer or invocation that was also a teaching spoken for me.

"Ayahuasca holds the key to the secrets of the jungle," he said. "Made and administered by a gifted shaman, with the grace of the spirits, ayahuasca can heal others, and unlock the mysteries of life."

When the sacred brew was ready many hours later, we doused the fire to let it cool. Then we lay in the hammocks in the hut for an early evening nap, taken as preparation for the exhausting, all-night ayahuasca healing ceremony still to come. When we woke, I was as rested and ready as I could be, though I wasn't looking forward to the repeated bouts of vomiting and diarrhea, the dreaded purging of stomach and intestines that ayahuasca induces, along with the much-desired visions.

"The *purga* of all the rot inside you, physical and emotional, is an important part of the healing," reminded don Antonio. "I've even added a few extra purgative plants into the medicine," he said with pride. "It is good for you!"

I knew he was right. The purga, unpleasant as it is, is an integral part of the healing experience. The tricky part of these repeated purgings is maintaining hygiene in the pitch-dark jungle, in the middle of the night, while "communing with the spirits" under the intoxicating effects of this unearthly vine.

I felt the characteristic pre-ceremony fears. Ayahuasca experiences are always intense, physically and emotionally, no matter how many times you imbibed. They are revelations delivered with a jackhammer. Don Antonio's stern admonitions today were an added weight on my mind and heart. I felt that he was preparing me for some difficult rite of passage, and that I stood forewarned.

My previous experiences with ayahuasca had been manageable at worst and ecstatic at best. I knew tonight would be different. To prepare myself, I began to "slow down," relaxing my body and quieting my mind. My mounting fear forced me to resort to every practice and principle don Antonio had taught me. Humility and reverence before the vine and its spirits was essential, and a healthy apprehension was unavoidable. I approached the ayahuasca spirits with a kind of half-dread half-faith, respecting their power, and yet open to their guidance and help. And I knew that I needed all the help I could get.

The healing ceremony began at 9 P.M. in front of the secluded hut in the pitch-dark jungle. First don Antonio invoked the spirits by singing his haunting ícaros. Between songs, he lit a pipe and repeatedly blew tobacco smoke, the shaman's breath, over the Medicine, now in a bottle, that we'd spent a long day making. After ritually blessing the Medicine, he turned and performed the same ritual blessing on me, alternately bathing me in tobacco smoke and singing ícaros.

The tobacco smoke enveloped me and the sacred ícaros entered my ears and vibrated deep within me. Each note he sang now seemed to vibrate with an ecstatic energy that reverberated in the cells of my body. All the fear and anxiety of the day gave way to a blissful peace. I felt the presence of spirit and I relaxed and opened to receive it. I had entered an altered state even before we drank the Medicine.

Then don Antonio poured into a calabash bowl a dose of thick, brown, chocolatey liquid—the residue of seven plants boiled in a clay pot for twelve hours. He offered more ícaros, smoke, and specific prayers over the sacred Medicine in the bowl, then he offered it to me to drink. I gagged down all at once my dose of the sweetish, sickening sludge. Immediately my insides "remembered" the taste, and wanted to vomit it up. While I choked back the urge, talking myself through these first few minutes of distress, don Antonio calmly drank his dose. Finally my body accepted the Medicine and I sat back and let it work on me.

About twenty minutes into the experience the purga began. For the next half-hour I was preoccupied with uncomfortable bodily functions, tending to them as best I could. The Medicine was definitely taking effect, yet I felt remarkably present and grounded. At one point, I lifted my head from a bout of vomiting, and in the peculiar luminosity ayahuasca imparts even to the darkness, I saw a large animal moving behind the trees, perhaps ten yards away. I froze involuntarily. Was it real or an effect of the Medicine? With ayahuasca, it can be hard to tell, the hallucinations are so real. There…it moved again. I focused my eyes intently on the large creature that, real or not, was coming toward us through the trees. Then, onto the path leading to the shaman's hut stepped a huge jaguar.

The enormous cat sauntered closer, seeming unaware of our presence. Then, when it was nearly 20 feet away, it looked up, right at me. The jaguar and I were both frozen now, eyes locked. The creature was stunningly beautiful, and easily weighed 250 pounds. In the ayahuasca light I saw its muscular body covered with golden brown fur dotted with large black rosette spots, with lighter yellow-gold patches on its chest and face.

I glanced over to where don Antonio had been moments before...he was gone. Out of the corner of my eye I saw him purging himself five yards away in the foliage. I looked back at the jaguar just as it sprang with a growl, fierce jaws wide open, fangs bared. I watched, still frozen, unable to cry out. "I'm dead...we're dead..." flashed through my mind, followed by the most intense, and unusual prayer I have ever prayed.

"If the shamans and their spirits have any power to protect me, let them show it now. If not, go ahead and eat me if you must."

Like a gazelle whose throat is already in the lion's jaws, I surrendered to my fate. And the most startling thing occurred. The jaguar closed its mouth, seemed to stop in mid-air, and fell quietly to the ground in front of me. Now, docile as a kitten, it started sniffing the ground as if it had lost my scent, seeming oblivious to me right in front of it. A few moments later it lost interest, wandered back into the jungle, and was swallowed up in darkness.

Don Antonio, seemingly out of nowhere, approached me with another bowl of Medicine, round two. Shaking uncontrollably, I pointed a trembling finger to the empty path where the jaguar had landed. "Did you see that?!" I asked him.

"What?" asked don Antonio.

"The jaguar!"

When I told him what I had seen, he said, "That was the ayahuasca testing you by taking you to your death. You could have died. You have done well." He nodded approvingly, "You have now taken on the spirit of the jaguar, and become the jaguar yourself. The fierceness and strength of your new jaguar spirit will protect you."

"More?" he asked, shoving another bowl of sickeningly sweet-smelling brew under my nose. Emotionally exhausted and still shaking, I couldn't even hold the bowl. I politely declined, "No, thanks."

CHAPTER 7

SPIRIT DOCTORS

A year had passed since my last trip to the rainforest. When I had left after my last visit, don Antonio had told me, "Don't come back until you've had one year of continuous celibacy."

Courage was just one spiritual gift I had received after facing my deepest fears and my death in my last encounter with the Medicine. Now, after a year of faithful and difficult celibacy, I felt stronger in body, mind, and spirit than ever before. In fact, I almost felt supercharged, as if my conserved sexual energy had transmuted into greater physical, mental, and psychic energy. This is the purpose of celibacy in shamanism, as in other spiritual paths. And this new energy was exactly the fuel I needed to be able to continue my rigorous apprenticeship with don Antonio. I was ready to return.

What an interesting year it had been. On my last visit I had encountered don Antonio's sternness, the power of the Medicine spirits, and my own guilty conscience. All three had fueled my determination to live the disciplina my apprenticeship required. At times in those first few months after my return, I had cried and felt sorry for myself, doubted my path, been frustrated, angry and resentful, and even contemplated abandoning my apprenticeship and never going back to Peru again. Much of this intense emotion was due to all the pent up energy I felt...so much that at times I could hardly sit still.

Sex is a common method of discharging energy—physical, emotional, and psychic—that we are unable to conduct in more creative ways. When celibacy denies us this discharge, the energy can build to an almost unbearable intensity. It can be like sitting in a fire, until we learn to channel the energy into higher uses such as creativity, healing, spiritual practice, etc. This is the purpose of celibacy in all shamanic/religious paths. But for much of the past year I had felt like a backed-up furnace, overheated, at times ready to explode. And I still had a year to go!

"The deeper the commitment, the stronger the medicine," don Antonio had said. After committing two years of my life to extreme dietas and a year of celibacy, I wondered what "stronger medicine" was still to come, and whether I would be able to take it.

I left for Peru with the usual stopover in Miami to change

planes. While waiting in the Miami airport between flights, I struck up a conversation with Kay, a friendly American woman in her fifties who was also on her way to Iquitos. Kay had a passion for pottery, and had studied with indigenous potters in Ecuador twenty years before. But she had mostly given up her craft to become a respiratory therapist in the United States.

She also told me that a childhood bout with polio had left her lame in one leg, and that recurring bouts of post-polio syndrome over the past few years had left her exhausted and depleted. She was on her way to the Amazon's lush tropical jungles to find rest and rejuvenation. We sat together on the plane to continue our conversation. When I told her a little about my apprenticeship as a healer with don Antonio, she expressed a strong interest in spiritual healing. Then she asked me outright if she could come with me to meet don Antonio and perhaps get a healing herself. I told her we could consider it further in Iquitos.

When we arrived in Iquitos, we both checked into the El Dorado hotel, located near the Plaza de Armas in the center of town. That night, while dining in the hotel restaurant, we struck up a lively conversation with a Canadian woman, a high-spirited family therapist in her mid-forties named Marcie who told us she'd come to Peru in search of a "spiritual adventure." As we shared stories, Marcie revealed that she was also looking for ways to integrate spiritual perspectives into her personal and professional life.

To make a long story short, by the end of the evening we were comrades in adventure, and they were both asking me to let them meet don Antonio. I agreed, wondering what don Antonio would say when I showed up with two unexpected guests.

Our rapido wound along the Napo River, past the familiar, progressively rising skyline of foliage and trees, deeper into the primal jungle. I now knew the route by heart. Don Antonio met us at the docks near the camp, and did not seem surprised to see *Los Tres Mosqueteros*, as we were now calling our adventurous threesome. He told me later he had seen himself in a dream several weeks ago, performing a healing with three white women. But he hadn't known what the dream meant until we arrived that afternoon.

During these first several days near don Antonio's childhood village on the Yanayacu River, he put us all to work in the medicinal plant garden. I had grown to love this place like home, I accepted shamanism on its own terms, and don Antonio was now like family to me, a loving taskmaster of spirit. But all of this was new for Kay and Marcie.

Don Antonio had announced his requirements for our working with him on the first afternoon, when I explained to him Kay and Marcie's reasons for coming.

"If you want to work with me, I will need a little work from you," he said, mincing no words. "If you want the spirits of the jungle and its plants to provide some healing for you, you must provide something for them in return. Working with spirit is always a reciprocal arrangement."

The next morning he handed each of us, respectively, a wheelbarrow, a shovel, and a machete for our first full day's work. His own trusty machete, as always, hung loosely in the belt around his waist.

"Tilling the soil is tilling your substance, too," he said. He pointed to a newly cleared section of land. "Prepare the land there to accept the new plant seeds I have collected from the jungle." He handed me a calabash full of tiny black seeds. "Connie will show you what to do," Then he added, "The jungle itself will prepare you and humble you."

Then he turned and walked off to work in another part of the gardens.

Yes, there is nothing like the jungle's intense heat, pesky mosquitoes, and non-stop tickling sweat to wear you down. The jungle *is* the medicine—to merely show up in the jungle guarantees a confrontation. And performing intense physical labor there forces a deeper level of surrender. This was no tourist expedition from the safety of a boat or cleared jungle path. This would be a dirty-up-to-the-elbows, sing-for-your-supper complete immersion experience. I wondered how Kay and Marcie would take to it.

In the first few days of work in the gardens, full of grumbling and sore muscles, Marcie and Kay began to fall into the rhythm of the jungle. The animal sounds, the afternoon rains, the spectacular beauty of the flora and fauna all worked its magic and medicine upon them. As the week wore on, we began to fall into rhythm with each other. Working together gave us an opportunity to talk at a deeper level and get to know each other better. Marcie and Kay got to know don Antonio better, too. And after each hard day's work, a limpia at dusk in a nearby stream with don Antonio deepened their connection to him. And after our limpias by the river's edge at the end of the week, don Antonio spoke to us.

"I am pleased with your work," he announced. "The spirits told me in my dream that you would come for a healing. And now they have told me that you are both ready for that. Tomorrow night, if you are willing, there will be an all-night healing ceremony." Both Kay and Marcie expressed a strong desire to undergo the ceremony, which they knew would include drinking the Medicine. Don Antonio was pleased.

"To prepare yourselves, do not eat anything tomorrow and spend the day in silent communion with nature. Kay, this first healing is for you. We will all come prepared and drink ayahuasca together. Remember," he concluded, "healing is a community effort. There are no observers. We will all participate in Kay's healing."

The symptoms of Kay's recurring post-polio syndrome flare-ups included chronic fatigue, increasing motor difficulties, and pain in her lame left leg. Being a healthcare professional, she had tried every conventional treatment available. Now, having reached a dead end, she was willing to try anything...even the ayahuasca healing ceremony that shaman don Antonio was now preparing on her behalf.

Kay intuitively knew she needed a deeper healing than conventional medicine offered, and which it had already failed to provide. She needed to reach into the spiritual depths where both illness and healing have their roots. And while grateful and excited at being allowed to participate in this shamanic healing ritual with don Antonio, she also had a case of the jitters at the prospect of drinking ayahuasca, the sacred Medicine don Antonio and I had, through rituals and words, been preparing her to meet.

During the day of preparation and ceremonial fasting, my body and mind began quieting down. I chose to spend my reflecting time swaying lazily in the arms of nature in a hammock strung in the shade of the jungle foliage, between a breadfruit tree and a cocoa tree. Toward the end of the day the heat, the sense of weightlessness and the swaying, and the late afternoon shadows flickering across my half-closed eyes, lulled me into a deep, peaceful trance.

Early evening is the in-between time, the intersection of light and darkness when don Antonio says the spirits reveal themselves. Now, after a day of fasting, contemplation and invoking the spirits for the evening ceremony, I began to notice faint milky silhouettes in the play of the shadows, against a distant background of dark-green jungle foliage. Some soared amidst a group of hanging lianas, flickering in and out of visibility the way fireflies do. Was I dreaming? Imagining? Perceiving reality beyond my "normal" senses? It didn't matter. I wasn't concerned. Their simple presence felt comforting.

As the sun set, and the awaited ayahuasca hour approached, I experienced the familiar pre-Medicine tension, a mixture of anticipation, excitement, anxiety, fear of the unknown, and a peculiar heightening of the senses, almost like a shadow cast by the Medicine's approach. I was soon drenched in sweat. My body/mind, as an *ayahuasquerita* (apprentice-in-training), always feels this peculiar anticipatory dread and respect which the Medicine commands. Ayahuasca healing ceremonies are intense ordeals on every level, physical, mental, emotional, and spiritual. Like the jungle itself, they are not for the faint of heart.

We were to meet don Antonio at the ceremonial hut at 9 P.M. sharp. At 8:30 P.M. we gathered in my room, said a last round of prayers together, and started down the path away from the camp toward don Antonio's ceremonial hut in the depths of the jungle. The sky was cloudy and the night was dark. Our ears rang with the nocturnal cacophony, the cries of animals searching for food, calling for mates, or simply bursting with the sheer, primal intensity of the jungle life force. I heard far off the powerful, unmistakable growl of a jaguar announcing an evening's hunt, and the disturbing phrase "eat or be eaten" popped uninvited into my mind.

As we walked along the path, the pitch dark jungle night

seemed to absorb our flashlight beams the way black holes are said to devour the light of stars. Somehow we lost our way…the slippery clay path turned to mud, then to an ankle-deep swamp, and we soon found ourselves floundering, legs tangled in the thickly growing camu camu plants that thrive in these common low-lying swamps. We walked in circles, bumping into each other, seeking a way out of the watery bog. The *Tres Mosqueteros* had become the *Tres Stooges*. I didn't know whether to laugh, cry, or scream for help.

Finally, not far off through the foliage, I spotted the candlelight that marked the shaman's hut. We moved directly toward it and soon reached the hut, our boots and feet drenched in a baptism-by-bog.

Don Antonio was there to welcome us. He wore his black ritual cushma, a jaguar tooth necklace, and his eyes already had the faraway look of one in touch with the spirit realm. He invited us to sit on the logs that formed a ceremonial circle in front of the hut. In the middle of the circle was a splendid table altar, his holy *mesa*. Lit candles formed a numinous ring around the table's edge, interspersed with boughs of healing plants. The candles represented our prayers and intentions for healing. In tonight's ceremony we would ask the spirits of the higher realms to heal us of things for which we had found no cures in the human realm.

"The spirits are already present around us," he said softly.

His statement immediately deepened the mood of our group. It often seems that our plight on Earth is to suffer the bondage of self—in troubles manifesting as physical, emotional, or spiritual afflictions—until death, the great purga, takes us into the beyond. We three had come far, at great expense and through much hardship, to reach this place in our lives, to attend this healing ceremony, to pray to unseen forces beyond our known reality for divine healing. Our allies in tonight's journey into the spirit realm sat in the center of the mesa, two hand-carved balsa figurines, a jaguar and anaconda—el tigre and el serpiente—and between them a dried piece of brown gnarled serpentine vine—ayahuasca. Don Antonio's shamanic healing tools—the tobacco, ayahuasca brew, bowls of perfume, and camphor water (for protection, don Antonio explained)—also sat on the table.

"Tonight," don Antonio began, "we will call on three friends and allies, three fearsome entities—the jaguar, the anaconda, and ayahuasca—for their great healing powers."

After briefly instructing Kay and Marcie regarding the ayahuasca experience and the formalities of the healing ceremony, he offered prayers and requests to the spirits of the heavens on our, and his behalf. As ayahuasca ceremonies are performed in complete darkness, he extinguished the candles, welcoming the spirits closer, then poured us each our dose of Medicine. We drank it in turn, managed to hold it down, and settled back to await its effects.

We occupied ourselves by wiping away the rivulets of sweat pouring down our faces, and waving our arms to chase away the ever-present swarms of mosquitoes that were eating us alive.

What an ordeal these jungle night ceremonies can be! Yet the outer jungle discomforts soon give way to internal phenomena of another order—dizziness, purging, visions, and altered states—as the Medicine takes effect. Then one finds oneself in a completely expanded and fluid dimension where normal limits on reality do not hold. This is the place where healings occur.

As I sat there feeling these multi-dimensional effects,

two luminous apparitions, a man and a woman, walked out of the velvety darkness of the jungle and stepped into our circle. Their bodies were almost like living X-rays, not quite skeletal, not flesh and blood, but glowing, three-dimensional entities distinctly human in size and shape. Oddly, they wore Western medical garb and comported themselves almost matter-of-factly, like ordinary physicians. Their faces were devoid of all expression, as if they were above human emotion. I knew that they were not humans, but spirit doctors, the healing spirits we had ritually invoked at the beginning of the ceremony.

Nothing in my previous ayahuasca journeys had prepared me for this extraordinary encounter. They stood in the ceremonial circle and I watched them, heart pounding.

I looked for don Antonio but he was no longer beside us. Then I looked around, straining my eyes in the darkness. He stood in the clearing amidst a swarm of bright yellowish orange dots. Face turned skyward, he waved his arms like a maestro in beautiful rhythmic gestures, conducting a ballet of fireflies and clouds.

The shaman was in his element, in deep communion with the spirits and full of ecstatic power, seeming both surrendered and very much in control. I saw that I was on my own. I could feel my heartbeat in my throat. My body was in a state of hyper-vigilance beyond the typical physiological effects of the Medicine.

It was time for a reality check. Focusing intently, I scanned my surroundings as best as I could in the dark to compare these two spirit apparitions with what I knew to be tangible realities. I saw: Kay and Marcie on their benches, retching on the ground, oblivious to our two luminous guests; the mesa in front of me; the hut; and the two spirit doctors.

All seemed equal, reality and spirit were indistinguishable to my present perceptions. This fact, both frightening and fascinating, was wreaking havoc with my sense of reality. I felt no fear of the spirit entities, who seemed benignly intent on their own purpose.

They went up to Kay, to whose healing this ceremony was primarily dedicated, and for whom we had invoked these spirits. I assumed they would work on Kay's left polio-stricken leg. Instead, to my puzzlement, they went behind her and stood looking intently at her back. "No...what are they doing?" I protested silently. "Can't they see that her leg is the problem?" I wondered again if this was a mere drug-induced hallucination.

I didn't have the confidence or presence of mind to speak to these spirit doctors and ask them what they were doing. Silent, I watched the event unfold. The male spirit now produced out of nowhere a glowing white globe of energy about the size of a bowling ball. He and the female spirit together held this ball of white light directly against Kay's spine at the base of her neck, then began to move it very slowly down her spine. After what seemed like an hour, they finally reached Kay's sacrum with the glowing ball and held it there for some time. Then, in an instant, they vanished.

Now I looked over and saw Marcie, lying on the ground in fetal position, moaning, clutching her head and her stomach, so ill she could not sit up. The Medicine does that sometimes. Don Antonio now came and knelt beside her and began working with her. He was still attending to her when Kay and I finally stumbled back to our rooms many hours later, and he continued attending to her through the night and into the morning.

I was disappointed by the spirit doctors' failure to treat

Kay's stricken leg, and by Marcie's prolonged ordeal with the Medicine. I had hoped they would both have a strongly positive experience. But this apparently had not occurred.

In the morning I crawled from under my mosquito net, still weak from the previous night's ceremony. Seeing Kay refilling her canteen at the water jug, I went and joined her, to rinse the putrid taste from my mouth and check in on her and see how she was feeling.

"Well," she asked me hopefully, "did you see me get a healing last night?"

I swished some water around in my mouth, trying to find a diplomatic answer, since I believed she hadn't received the healing she so desired. If I was disappointed, I knew she would be also. I felt responsible for her experience, and guilty that I had enthusiastically recounted to Kay, days earlier, several extraordinary ayahuasca healing stories. I felt I had given her false hope.

"Well, umm, I don't know, Kay," I began. "I'll just tell you what I saw."

I then told her how two spirit doctors had come to her out of the jungle, pressed a bright ball of light against her spine for some time, running it from her neck down to her sacrum, and after leaving it there a while, had suddenly vanished. I didn't mention their glaring omission…they had ignored her leg. I was surprised when Kay lit up at my report with a huge smile. She noticed my puzzled look.

"Don't you get it, Connie?" she said. "Do you remember the etiology of polio? The virus attacks the motor neurons of the spinal cord. The polio-damaged motor-neurons in my spine that were still functioning are now failing me. That's what post-polio syndrome is." She was quite excited. "Those spirit doctors went right to the source of the problem. It sounds like they were recharging my failing spinal motor-neurons with that glowing ball of energy."

This struck me as utterly remarkable. I had paid little attention to polio as a healthcare professional…it had essentially been eradicated in the United States before I reached pharmacy school. I now realized the misunderstanding had been mine. I was expecting them to treat the branches, while they had gone straight to the root of the problem. Had they merely treated Kay's leg as I had expected them to do, they would have ignored the real problem, the damaged motor-neurons in the spine which were responsible for her post-polio disintegration.

When I asked her what she had experienced, she made the following report.

"I saw a golden ball of light moving toward my body and stop still in front of me. I gazed at its inviting glow and saw my life bathed in a new light. As I continued staring at the golden light, I saw pieces of my life rearrange themselves. I realized that I was working too hard in a job that was not my true calling. When I was thinking about my job, the light grew dimmer. When I thought about my life continuing as it is, into the future, the light was nearly extinguished. When I thought about my real passion for making Ecuadorian pottery, the golden light grew bright and intense, and it made me feel warm, loved, connected, and ecstatically happy. I feel physically and emotionally energized right now, even though I feel like I should rest."

This seeming contradiction between my perception of what had happened, and Kay's reported experience, showed me both the mysterious power of the Medicine as well as my continuing inclination to "separate" mind and body. Our conversation helped me to realize that both the body and spirit healing of a patient are always going on at the same time; they are not separate. I learned that whether I am aware of them or not, there are many levels of an integrating healing happening at once, to ultimately make "whole" the patient.

We all spent the day recuperating, quietly reflecting, taking naps to recharge and catch up on the sleep we'd missed during the all-night ceremony. Yet despite the intense nature of ayahuasca, it does not wear the body down. In all, ayahuasca is profoundly healing and rejuvenating. Not only do I feel a greater sense of energy and aliveness over time, I also feel calmer and more grounded because of it as well. That is one reason it is called the Medicine. Late that afternoon don Antonio came into my room off the maloca and announced an ayahuasca healing ceremony to be held the next evening for Marcie. When he left I moaned and rolled over on my cot, wondering if I could really go through this again so soon. Still recuperating, I felt physically spent, emotionally drained, and my mind was in shreds.

"Well, you can be a shamana," I reminded myself, "or go back to pharmacy."

Neither option seemed particularly appealing at the moment. It took what little energy I had left to crawl from under my mosquito netting and grab some dinner. After that I went straight back to bed again. I would need all my strength for tomorrow evening's ceremony.

At 9 P.M. the next evening, after another day's fast, we were again seated on the logs of the ceremonial circle outside the shaman's hut, as prepared as we could be for the long night ahead. The smell of the burning copal, an aromatic jungle tree resin, on the mesa helped us to turn our focus inward to our intentions for the night. Don Antonio finished his preparations and blessed each of us with songs and tobacco smoke, covering Marcie in a blue swirling cloud. Marcie, the focus of tonight's ceremony, had no physical maladies or complaints. I wondered what she might need besides a general healing and a spiritual blessing.

After the ritual blessing, don Antonio offered us each a dose of the Medicine and we settled in to wait. The sky was clear tonight and the light of the full moon radiated through the jungle canopy, pouring down through the clearing over the ceremonial area. This would make it easier to navigate back and forth when the purga began. And begin it did…soon we were taking turns vomiting into the bushes. After this subsided, my mind cleared and my senses sharpened.

Forty-five minutes into the ceremony, I saw a far-off glow in the jungle, steadily approaching. As it drew nearer I made out the two spirit doctors. They had come again. They walked straight to Marcie and began a formal, even clinical examination. They first lifted her T-shirt and took turns palpating her stomach. Each carefully pressed and felt all around her abdominal area, as any Western physician might do. Marcie seemed oblivious to their presence. Don Antonio was sitting on his log, looking elsewhere, absorbed in his own experience, seeming unaware of what I was seeing.

Tonight I was determined to speak with the spirit doctors, to interact with and learn from them. So I asked them if they were teaching me how to palpate patients. When they didn't respond, I reached over to Marcie and put my hands directly on top of theirs, thinking to learn their technique.

"No," the female spirit doctor clearly said. "You don't do anything. We do all the work. You just host the vision."

Having been given my place, there was nothing to do but sit back and watch them work. Next they lowered Marcie's pants and took turns palpating her pelvic area, from left to right, slowly, intently, with great care. Then I noticed them focusing on Marcie's left pelvic area. After spending a good deal of time there, they stopped to converse in undertones. The female spirit doctor seemed quite concerned. She pressed deeply several times on one particular spot on Marcie's left pelvic side. Each time Marcie would clutch her abdomen, groan, and then vomit. But she still seemed unaware of the two entities working on her.

Then, to my utter surprise, the female spirit doctor looked up at me and said, "She has ovarian problems."

"Are you sure?" I asked. "She hasn't complained or said anything about it."

"We are sure," she replied.

"What should I do about it?" I was feeling very troubled and at a loss.

"*You* don't do anything about it," the spirit doctor said, reminding me of who has the real power here. "We will take care of her. We are going to perform surgery."

Riveted, I sat on my log and watched fascinated while the spirit doctors performed some sort of operation on Marcie's ovaries. They both bent over her, focused intently on her pelvic area. One of them held Marcie's clothing out of the way while the other moved both hands over Marcie's ovaries. I was unable to distinguish exactly what was being done, but it seemed effortless and was over soon. When they had finished the procedure, Marcie's vomiting episodes had subsided. Then, in silence, the spirit doctors walked off into the jungle from whence they came.

Again, once they had disappeared I immediately began doubting what I'd seen. I looked over at Kay and don Antonio for confirmation, but they were both busy retching by the side of the hut. Marcie, her "surgery" finished, lay exhausted on the ground. I still didn't know what to think or believe. I decided to talk to don Antonio in the morning about my "vision."

In the early morning hours, exhausted by the Medicine and the night's events, I climbed into the hammock inside the hut and fell into a deep sleep. When I woke the next morning, Kay, Marcie, and don Antonio were gathered out front around the mesa for a ceremonial closing circle, a kind of group debriefing. Kay would do the translating for us. Don Antonio had made everyone a tall glass of *limón* water, with jungle lime, a post-ayahuasca morning tonic. Don Antonio nodded to me as I joined in, and then toasted the group.

"*Salud*, to your health, " he raised his glass and sipped the tart green limewater. He began with a heartfelt acknowledgment, and then got to the point. "Marcie, I'll start with you. First, I want to thank you for the sacrifices of time and energy you made to come here and participate in this healing ceremony. Now I must tell you something. I'm afraid that you have ovarian problems."

Marcie's eyes showed fearful concern. I was dumbstruck. Don Antonio's words seemed to corroborate my vision of the previous night. I had spoken to no one, had told no one what I had seen, and believed that only I knew what had transpired during last night's healing ceremony. Had don Antonio also seen the spirit doctors? Had we entered the same healing realm together last night? Could I, as his apprentice, now access the spirit realms where this healing work was done?

"What does that mean?" asked Marcie. "What should I do?"

"Don't worry," said don Antonio, gently patting her shoulder. "The spirit doctors performed spiritual surgery on you last night during the ceremony."

My god! I thought. *They're real!* Apparently I wasn't the only one who saw the spirit doctors last night, who heard their diagnosis and witnessed the "surgery." This was the confirmation I needed. Now I could finally believe my own eyes. The spirit realm was real.

Meanwhile, Marcie looked relieved, even radiant. The color returned to her face and she said, "That's interesting...you see, I had ovarian surgery as an adolescent. When my mother was pregnant with me she took the hormone DES, diethylstilbesterol, and it screwed up my ovaries. It didn't occur to me to tell you about it, since it happened so long ago. I thought I was done with all that.

"I was so sick last night," she continued. "Sick to death of myself. I've always felt ashamed that I couldn't have children, that I'm no good for any man. I've run away from every meaningful relationship I've ever had. But I feel like I've purged all the shame from my body somehow. I don't feel defective right now. I feel lovable."

Being a pharmacist, I knew the daughters of women who took the hormone diethylstilbesterol during their pregnancies suffered many reproductive problems as a result. Marcie's story further corroborated my experience with the spirit doctors, and the accuracy of their diagnoses. And it implied that a deeper spiritual healing, which Western medicine did not offer, was still needed some thirty years later.

"This is the start of a healing process for both of you,"

replied don Antonio, looking at Marcie, and then at Kay. "But it's up to you to make this a turning point. This is not a magical ceremony that removes a lifetime of physical distress. Even when spirit heals, you must still do your part afterwards, and make necessary life-adjustments and changes. Otherwise you may simply reproduce further illness later on. This is how it is. You must follow the rest of the prescription, or you may lose what you have gained here."

Now he looked at Kay. "Spirit showed you that you must stop working full-time at your job," he said. "It is robbing you of vital energy you need to heal. Use the extra time you have to do what you really love, something that makes you feel good. Spirit has given you much healing energy with the limpias, the ícaros, and the ayahuasca. Now you must generate your own energía positiva for your ongoing healing."

Kay's eyes lit up as she quickly answered him. "Making pottery is the passion of my life. But I haven't had the time or energy to do it for years. I'm afraid that if I don't work, I won't have enough money to take care of myself because of my deteriorating health."

"My dear lady," don Antonio replied firmly, "if you don't stop working so hard, you won't have a life worth saving. You are killing yourself slowly. But it's your life!"

I could see that Kay took his words seriously. She knew in her heart that he was right. And she now promised to act on his words when she got home. Now don Antonio turned his attention to Marcie, who nervously awaited his "prescription."

"Marcie, you must find yourself a good man and settle down. I can see in your heart how unsettled and out of balance you have been. Your sexuality is in chaos." Don Antonio sipped his lime drink and waited.

"You're right," said Marcie. "My relationships have always been confused and fleeting. I never realized how much it had to do with my DES condition."

"Our physical health reflects our spiritual and emotional health," don Antonio said. "Mind, body, and emotions are interconnected. A shaman never treats the body as separate from the whole being. What you have experienced here is a start. You have a deep wound. Find a healing relationship. Listen to your spirit. And find a shaman in your area who can continue this work with you. I recommend daily treatments of healing limpias and ícaros for a month."

Marcie looked down at the ground. "We don't have many shamans where I live. I'm not sure I'll be able to find one."

"Connie can continue this work with both of you long-distance. The spirits will come to her in dreams to help her assist you. It is better in person, but it can also be done from far away. She is ready to give healings and will be helping many others in her country. The spirits are around her."

I took a sip of lime drink and stared deeply into the green liquid. A mysterious medicinal world in microcosm seemed to swirl, with bits of lime, in my glass. Now I told don Antonio of my ayahuasca experiences with the spirit doctors, how I had spoken with them and watched them perform spiritual surgery on Marcie's ovaries. I asked him to explain what it all meant, and what part he played in the healing ceremony.

"You could say the shaman is the doctor, the surgeon, and the ayahuasca is an x-ray machine and a scalpel," don Antonio began. "The scalpel does not perform the surgery without the doctor. Patients do not perform surgery on themselves. And no one should drink ayahuasca without a shaman's guidance. The shaman and the Medicine should go hand in hand."

"So who were the spirit doctors I saw?" I asked.

"They were the spirits of the ayahuasca who help shamans. The patient drinks the ayahuasca in order to open up to the actions of these spirit doctors, whom they do not see. I can invoke and work with the spirit doctors because I have become one with the Medicine. Now you see them, because through your apprenticeship with the spirit and power of ayahuasca, you are also becoming one with the Medicine. This is what it means to be a shaman."

"As a shaman gains his powers, he is able to see inside people and make a diagnosis anytime it is needed, even without the assistance of ayahuasca. Limpias and ícaros performed by a shaman can heal the same as drinking the Medicine. A shaman may give a patient medicinal plants, to be taken internally, or applied externally; or, he may give a patient magical plants that open him to the spirit realms. It depends on which is needed. Yet medicinal plants, or magical plants...it's all the same in the end. It's all the healing power of spirit in jungle medicine."

CHAPTER 8

THE SHAMAN
AND THE
SURGEON

A t the end of our debriefing ceremony, don Antonio prescribed a thirty-day period of celibacy for Kay and Marcie. All who drink ayahuasca with don Antonio receive these same instructions, with sometimes further restrictions recommended. Disciplinas are an integral means of continu-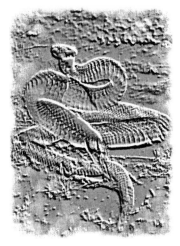ing the healing process and enhancing the spiritual benefits of the ceremony, a way of fully receiving ayahuasca's gifts and allowing the Medicine to continue working on one with as little interference as possible.

"It is not enough just to drink the Medicine," don Antonio explained to the two women who were about to return home. "You must continue to cooperate with it after the ceremony ends. It is still working in you, trying to help you. But if you dissipate its healing energy through sex, you have wasted your time and mine."

They both gave me a questioning look, and I nodded with the authority of my own experience in trying to skirt this particular rule. Personal responsibility for one's own healing process is a significant principle in jungle shamanism. No cooperation, no blessings.

"In order to heal people, three things must be present," don Antonio had instructed me early on. "They must believe in your medicine. They must want to heal. And they must follow directions."

Irresponsibly refusing to cooperate with the healing process—as by continuing destructive behavior and relationships—is endemic in the West. No doctor and no medicine can make up for non-cooperation on the part of the patient. Don Antonio was right. The patient must want to heal, believe in the medicine, follow directions, and take full responsibility for that essential part of the healing process which they alone can fulfill.

What good does it do to drink ayahuasca, or take remedial medication, and then continue a way of living that is the source of your health problems? Healing is an on-going cooperative effort, a relationship between patient and healer, and patient with her/himself, and with the life-force that is spirit. There must be mutual respect among all parties. The healing process must receive its due in order to fulfill its promise. Don Antonio is a hard taskmaster precisely because of his understanding of and commitment to this vision of healing.

I saw how deeply affected Kay and Marcie were by their experiences and by don Antonio's efforts on their behalf. They seemed committed to carrying out his directions, even in their busy modern lives back home. They stayed on for another week, working in the gardens, absorbing the "medicine" of the jungle, and trying to integrate their experiences as much as possible before returning home.

One week after their healings, they bid don Antonio and I goodbye and returned to the United States, enriched by their time in the rainforest. I stayed behind for several more days to continue my work with don Antonio. A quiet fell over the camp as we began preparing for one final ayahuasca ceremony before my departure.

I had learned much from the past two years of disciplinas and ceremonies. Last week I had reached another level of my shamanic apprenticeship. I had been opened into direct contact with the spirit doctors, and played a shamana's role— the "host," as the spirit doctors had said—in Marcie and Kay's healing ceremony.

Now, two evenings after Marcie and Kay's departure, don Antonio and I stood alone in the ceremonial circle, before the candle-lit mesa outside his jungle hut. He graciously motioned for me to take a seat on one of the logs.

"Shamanism is a life-long commitment, Connie," he began. "Now you have lived the arduous disciplinas and dietas and the spirits recognize your commitment. They have responded by appearing to you and treating your first patients. *Es un buen símbolo.* This is a good sign. They are pleased. And I am pleased. You have passed this test. You are now ready for more."

He bent his head, lit his ceremonial tobacco, paused and then looked up at me. "You are like this dry tobacco," he said, "and I am the burning match. I have kindled a flame within you. Now you are responsible for that flame. It is time to commit yourself fully to spirit, not just to me and to learn and obey its teachings and *disciplinas*, not just mine."

He took a long drag on his cigarette and spewed the shaman's breath—clouds of tobacco smoke—all over me. My consciousness began shifting as don Antonio began singing ícaros and rhythmically tapping my body with his shacapa. The whirling smoke and hypnotic rhythms of his chants and rattling leaves pushed me into a deep trance.

Don Antonio paused to sip some water. Then he said, "I am singing new songs, more ícaros, into you tonight. Like seeds, they will grow inside of you over time. All things of great value take time. *Paciencia*, be patient, my friend. It is a lifetime of commitment and learning."

He began singing again, mesmerizing songs that drew me into a most profound state of relaxation. I had given up wondering about or trying to explain these states. Don Antonio's *"es magia,* (it's magic)," seemed as good an explanation as any. Now I simply accepted these experiences as forms of spirit.

Then don Antonio and I each swallowed a calabash full of ayahuasca and sat back to wait for the shift of consciousness. The two recent ayahuasca healings had softened and macerated me. A level of resistance I'd always felt waiting for the Medicine to take effect, was gone. I felt more open than ever before to the guidance of spirit.

Now the shift into ayahuasca consciousness began. My body and mind, and my presumed knowledge about "the way things really are," seemed to melt away, and I felt I myself slipping into a realm of universal consciousness, of all possibilities, into reality where we can all be healed and whole.

Surrendered to this process, my spirit soared to the chartless expanse of the inner universe, along a path taken by all true shamans before me.

It wasn't long before the spirit doctors arrived. There was no surprise in me this time. They stood before me, giving me their full attention. Then the male spirit doctor leaned over me, reached down and touched my throat, and began to carefully examine the scar area where my thyroid surgery had taken place three years ago. The female spirit doctor asked me to lean my head back a bit to make the examination easier. I obliged, and the two of them continued.

Now comfortable communicating with these entities, I struck up a natural conversation with them. "Thank you for checking me over and looking into my health," I told them gratefully. "I really appreciate it." Then I reflected on how it felt to be a cancer survivor, living with the dread of recurrence always in the back of my mind. "Will it come back?" is a fear most cancer survivors carry with them. Now I asked the spirit doctors examining my throat what I would ask any doctor in this circumstance.

"How is my throat? Am I still cancer-free?"

"Yes, you're doing just fine there," the female spirit doctor answered. "But that's not why we're here." She paused a moment and I looked at her directly. Then she announced, *"We've come to give you your voice."*

With that, they both put their hands on my neck. My throat seemed to open wider and wider, until it felt like a giant church organ pipe, ready to express the divine music of life. Now powerful sacred healing songs, the ícaros, spontaneously welled up from deep inside me, billowing into my newly-opened throat, pouring out in a beautiful melodious chanting. Eyes closed, I sang from every pore in my body a

159

melody I had never heard before. I'm not a singer; normally I can't carry a tune. But this was truly beautiful. I looked to the spirit doctors, wondering where this magical song was coming from. But they had vanished.

At that point, don Antonio leaned over and told me to quiet down, like a patient father gently chastising his child. He preferred his healing ceremonies to be quiet, controlled and internally focussed. I struggled to turn off the music now ringing in every cell of my body from some "all-shaman's" radio station in the spirit realm. But I could not silence it. With great effort, I managed to muffle myself for a few strained moments. But the sweet notes continually bubbled up from within. And soon the lyrical ícaros came floating out of my throat again. Don Antonio now realized what was happening.

"Ah, the ícaros!" he exclaimed, breaking his own rule of silence. "Sing, my dear, sing," he said, now repeatedly swooping his arms up from his waist, palms upturned, as if to encourage the notes within me.

The songs poured out of me, off and on through the entire ceremony. Not being musical, I'd never really understood what the ícaros were about. I knew that gurus, priests, and shamans of many cultures chanted and sang songs with entrancing, spellbinding power to heal the sick and alter their consciousness. I had experienced this power personally in my work with don Antonio.

Yet though don Antonio had told me shamans were given the ícaros by spirit, I thought it was his lyrical way of saying they made them up (or learned them by rote from their teachers). Now I was being given these songs from within. I experienced them as a mysterious gift from a deep place revealed by the Medicine; a gift of spirit as don Antonio had said. Now I understood their healing power. An ícaro, like all divinely inspired music, is a bridge to the other realm. It comes through the shaman into this world. First it sings the shaman. Then the shaman sings the ícaro, and it connects him, and the one he sings to, to the place and power from whence it came.

You might say the concept of magical healing songs is as far from a pill in a bottle as Jesus Christ is from Isaac Newton. Both have their place, neither one necessarily cancels out the other, and the two together are better than either alone. In my case, the scientist who formerly dispensed pills in a bottle, became a singer dispensing spirit in a song. Becoming an open channel for spirit had made me, for the first time, an inspired pharmacist! And I marveled as these enchanted melodies floated out of me through the night into the wee hours of the morning.

I dozed and ate alternately throughout the next day, recouping lost sleep and nourishment. My daydreams and my dozing dreams were vivid, even lucid. In one dream I saw my throat, now completely opened, and understood the meaning of being "given my voice." It referred to the sacred songs that had come through me, and also to the inner freedom to speak my truth, to tell my personal vision, without fear of being labeled crazy—a fear instilled in me by my mother's tragic life, and carried with me ever since at great personal cost. I saw the "life of quiet desperation" I had lived since childhood—"quiet" for the reasons mentioned above, and "desperate" because of the hopelessness that living a false life begets.

In another important dream I saw my HMO clinic surgeon

removing a physical lump from my throat...my cancerous thyroid. Super-imposed on this scene, I saw the spirit doctors removing an energy block in my throat...my fear of speaking my truth. This revealing juxtaposition told me the tension/ block caused by this fear had constricted the life-force in my throat, resulting over time in my thyroid cancer.

I understood that for my own healing to be complete, I had needed the help of both technological *and* spiritual medicine. I was seeing that technology and spirit can coexist and collaborate, and that their integration is *necessary* for a truly modern holistic medicine to be achieved. In that moment, I knew the focus of my work as a pharmacist and a shamana was this integration of spirit and medicine, as both had played an integral part in my own spiritual and physical healing.

This last dream ended with both the surgeon and the sha- man, don Antonio, looking into my eyes at the same time. As I awoke, this image lingered briefly, then the surgeon's face disappeared. But don Antonio's face remained, staring down at me in my hammock. He had been quietly, patiently watch- ing me nap, knowing that spirit communicates much during these times.

In that moment, I felt profound gratitude for both the shaman and the surgeon, for spirit and the scalpel. I acknowl- edged the blessings of spirited medicine and technological medicine, each divinely conceived through man whether he knows it or not. I owed my life to both of them.

Around 8:30 P.M. I climbed through the mosquito net- ting into my bed and tucked myself in. I lay there, thinking about the spirit doctors, fascinated by their healing abilities, and amazed at their remarkable participation in the ceremonies. I felt that we were developing a working relationship. Yet I was puzzled as to who or what these entities actually were. *"Who are these spirit doctors?"* I kept thinking. And with this last question lingering in my mind, I drifted off to sleep.

In the middle of the night, the spirit doctors appeared to me in a dream as a mass of swirling energy.

"You called for us?" they asked, almost like genies summoned from a lamp.

"Yes," I answered. "I'm curious. Exactly who and what are you? How can I explain you to others?"

"We are the shear unbridled healing forces of nature that you, as a shamana, are learning to harness and call upon," they answered.

I first took this in relation to myself, and wondered if I was due a bit of credit for Kay and Marcie's healings. But they quickly spoke in answer to this unspoken thought.

"It is we, the generative forces of nature, who do the healing. Not you." And with that, they slipped away. And so did I, into the depths of a sound sleep.

It was time for me to go home. Don Antonio and I shared the first leg of the return journey, a long boat ride through the primal jungle towards civilization. He was going with me as far as Iquitos.

I planned to check in on Marcie and Kay in a few weeks, to see what effects their healings might be having over time.

After a while, I became aware of the hum of the boat's engine vibrating through the hull, and through my own body, lulling me into a pleasant trance. I sat quietly, looking out into the jungle—a mass of vegetation—simply feeling what was happening. I noticed my body swelling with the sound, as in previous ceremonies, and realized I was like an antenna picking up vibratory frequencies from the mass of vegetation that surrounded me, resonating to the primal sounds, the music and vibration of the rainforest.

In a kind of rapture, I looked up at don Antonio, caught his eye, and motioned to our surroundings.

"This jungle is in my body and in my blood," I said to him.

He gave a nod, surveying the lush panorama.

"Yes, I know," he said. "Me, too."

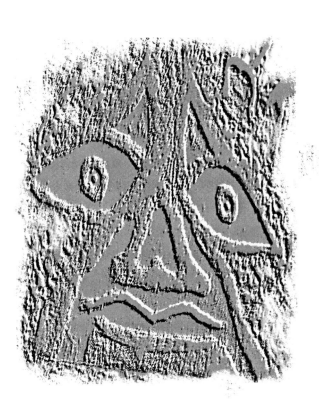

AMAZON REFLECTIONS

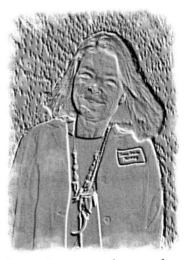

I n the Amazon rainforest I had experienced nature's healing power as a symphonic confluence of plant and Earth and spirit energies. If plants had a spiritual impact on humans, as well as an herbal/medicinal effect, then being in the rainforest was an immersion in a spiritual/ medicinal environment of immense healing power. This source of countless medicinal plants, known and yet to be discovered, was our planet's most potent natural medicine chest, and its most vibrant healing oasis.

My encounters with the spirit of the rainforest, in the

most intimate of communions, had charged me with a sense of urgency to do some kind of work on behalf of this threatened Eden. Both don Antonio and I share this common vision. We have dedicated our lives to the conservation of the Amazon rainforest, *la selva*, as well as to the continuation of the lineage of its shamanic practices. By conserving, or "serving with," the healing plants and healing traditions of the rainforest, we also serve ourselves. We are changed by actively participating in the conservation of these healing powers, this *jungle medicine*. In this process, we absorb the spirit we so desperately need in order to respirit our own lives—our people, our medicine, and our healers.

As don Antonio reminds all of us, it's a reciprocal arrangement; the more you commit, the stronger the spiritual reward. Our many projects for Amazonia's flora and fauna, its people and healing traditions we call 'The Spirit of La Selva'. You are invited to apprenticeship yourself to the spirit of the rainforest, to join us in our mission to conserve the healing powers of the rainforest.

And now, having returned from the rainforest, I settled back into the predatory jungle of modern Western life. I was eager to put to use what I had learned in the rainforest.

"Connie," don Antonio had said to me on my last visit. "Stay close to nature. Silence yourself and listen. The plants have secrets to tell you. They can help you and your patients. When a shaman wants to learn the medicinal properties of any plant, he asks the plant, then listens closely, and the information comes directly from the plant itself. Of course this is only the start. One must also test and experiment with the plant and prove its medicinal value. But a shaman can gain information in ways that other people overlook."

Years ago I had experienced this process of direct knowing don Antonio had described. First with the forget-me-nots. Later, I had seen the bristly bottle-brush horsetail one night in a dream, then in reality the next day, and it had cured my now ex-husband's bleeding bladder. I had also received information from, and felt the medicinal energetic effects of gingko and feverfew.

According to don Antonio, *asking* plants for information, and receiving it directly—either telepathically or by other remarkable means—was an ancient shamanic source of medicinal wisdom. This method also accounted for the shaman's spiritual relationship to medicinal plants, which don Antonio had often spoken of. And of course, a shaman's knowledgeable and effective use of herbs on a purely medicinal level was a litmus test of his or her legitimacy.

Now, reflecting on my experiences of the past several years, both during my shamanic apprenticeship under don Antonio, and in my work in Dr. Dee's natural medicine clinic, I began to ask myself, "What essential healing wisdom has been given to me that I can share with others?"

One afternoon several months after my return from Peru, my neighbor and friend Josie called, feeling depressed and needing someone to talk to. For the past few years Josie had experienced recurring bouts of mild to moderate depression. Her physician had prescribed a series of antidepressants that had given her little or no relief, and had even triggered a variety of unpleasant side-effects.

Six months earlier, deciding to wean herself from her pharmaceutical regime, Josie had come to see me to discuss "natural" alternative treatments. To a conventional pharmacist trained to view depression as an effect of faulty brain chemistry, balancing the brain's neurotransmitters through pharmaceutical intervention—a prescription antidepressant—would seem the logical treatment. Better living through modern chemistry.

By then, I was anything but a conventional pharmacist. I had recommended that Josie try St. John's Wort, clinically shown to be effective in cases of mild to moderate depression. Now, six months later, Josie told me she had taken St. John's Wort for three months with no benefit (and fortunately no side-effects). For the past three months she'd used no herbal or conventional medicines, having lost confidence in both. Yet she still felt that she needed something to help her with her depression.

Now, with a clearer understanding of my work with don Antonio than I had had six months ago, I began considering Josie's problem from a deeper perspective, as a spiritual condition. While waiting for Josie to arrive on my doorstep, I remembered don Antonio's admonition to me.

"Remember the plants, Connie," he had said. "And trust the spirits."

Over a cup of tea, Josie described her depression, with its cycles of anxiety, fatigue, hopelessness, and low self-esteem. As she talked, I simply listened with full attention. At one point, in my mind's eye, I had a faint impression of the spirit doctors leading her out into a field somewhere. I mentally noted the image. When she described not being able to muster enough energy to get out of bed in the morning, I felt an intuitive clarity about what she should do, guided by the inner image that had come to me.

I told Josie that she should get up early each morning, go outside, and spend time in nature. I encouraged her to volunteer in one the many gardens in the various retreat centers in our area, sensing that this might just be the field into which I had seen her being led. That was all the advice I gave her. I recommended no herbs or medications. I knew this was exactly the right "spiritual prescription."

Six weeks later Josie called again, this time excitedly. She'd been working as a volunteer gardener at a local meditation retreat center. On her first morning, the head gardener had assigned her to weed a huge unkempt bed of lavender. It had taken her six hours. Did the head gardener know that lavender is an herbal remedy, useful in treating some cases of anxiety and depression? Perhaps. But he hadn't known that Josie suffered from just these symptoms.

That day Josie was infused with lavender…its fragrance, its soothing colors, its medicinal essential oils, its spiritual essence. Six hours of smelling, touching, looking at and crawling through a bed of lavender, digging her hands in the earth and basking in the sun's energizing rays had let nature do its healing work. By the end of the day, she noticed that her anxiety and depression had markedly lifted.

Ecstatic over her change of mood, Josie had come home and "gone lavender." Her clothes, her perfume, the new color of her bedroom, she now told me excitedly, were all lavender. And besides doing ongoing work in the garden, she now pampered herself daily with lavender herbal baths. She hadn't been bogged down by depression lately, and she credited the lavender connection with her newfound sense of well being.

Her story seemed to confirm the healing spiritual influence of certain plants that don Antonio often spoke about. And the intuitive image of the spirit doctors leading Josie into a field that had come to me in our previous conversation now seemed more than mere coincidence. However these events had come about, it did seem that Josie had been led to her cure, and that nature, and spirit, deserved the credit for her healing.

"Josie, I owe you an apology," I said when she finished her story.

"What for?" she asked. "I'm grateful to you."

"In our first consultation six months ago I was still being a conventional pharmacist. I recommended the ingestion of an herbal medicine, but I was thinking pharmaceutically."

I now saw that in that first consultation, I hadn't comprehended that natural healing meant healing through the power of nature. I'd been locked into the conventional view that healing was an effect produced only by medicine taken orally or injected into the bloodstream. Now I saw that healing wasn't exclusively dependent on such literal processes. Conventional medical procedures, you could say, were like the letter of the law of healing. But there was also the spirit of law, which was the "ingestion" of spirit itself, whether the spirit of lavender, of nature, of a healer or saint, or of a life filled with meaning and purpose. Conventional medicine, it seemed to me, followed the letter of the law. Shamans, and all true healers, followed the spirit of the law. And both letter and spirit were needed for a truly holistic, or spirited medicine, to be achieved.

Josie, now bubbling effusively with "energia positiva," seemed revitalized. At the end of our conversation, I thanked her for the educational demonstration she had unwittingly given me, and hung up the phone, feeling like a novice all over again. I had learned once more what don Antonio had been saying in different ways from the beginning of my apprenticeship: *"The medicine is not in the pill. Only spirit heals."*

Another demonstration was right around the corner. One

afternoon, while leaving a natural products conference in San Francisco, I bumped into Dave, a successful entrepreneur who owned an herbal mail-order business. Actually, Dave bumped into me. Looking harried and preoccupied, he glanced up to apologize to whomever he'd nearly trampled in his mad rush from "here" to "there." We recognized each other and stopped to chat for a few minutes.

The herbal mail-order business was Dave's third or fourth business venture. Each of his previous ventures had made him a millionaire. Dave, a mega-success type A personality, was a man with a classic competitive drive. My impression was that no matter whom he was talking to or what the circumstance, he was always doing business. Only today his hyper monologue on herbal sales and marketing woes showed that he was clearly stressed and distressed. Just listening to him made me anxious.

The gist of it was worry...his sales were lagging, maybe he'd entered the herbal business too late, maybe this time he'd chosen the wrong business venture. I saw an herbal tycoon on a worry treadmill generating stress ulcers. He was wealthy enough that even the end of his catalogue would only be a minor financial setback. Yet he was still obsessing himself sick over his business.

I recalled the Dave of a year ago, a man so inspired by his own personal healing through herbs that he'd started an herbal remedy catalogue, hoping to succeed in a new business venture while doing the world some good.

"Have you run across any exciting new herbal remedies in your jungle adventures?" he now asked me, and added, "Like maybe a cure for ulcers?"

It seemed he was looking for something to save his business and his stomach.

Looking at his condition from my current perspective, it didn't seem far-fetched that Dave's business woes and his physical problems might be dual manifestations of a "spiritual" imbalance, a life-dilemma. A spirited medicine approached seemed in order, since even the best herbal remedy is no substitute for finding and addressing the root of a condition. Dave seemed willing to try just about anything. And I was willing to help. I had only experience and knowledge to gain, and nothing but a couple of hours to lose. I invited him to come home with me for a cup of tea and a shamanic healing. I would sing the healing ícaros to the rhythm of the shacapa over him, just as don Antonio had on me. I just trusted what I had been taught. He readily accepted.

Forty minutes later we were sipping a preliminary cup of tea in my living room. After tea, I had Dave sit on a dining room chair in the middle of the room. I took my Amazon shacapa in hand and began the ritual, tapping it rhythmically on his head. I glanced out my window at the beautiful passionflower vine growing up the neighbor's trellis, and a spontaneous ícaro, a new healing song, rose within me. I began singing softly, tapping the shacapa over Dave's body, around his shoulders, down his back, over his legs, down to his feet, several times. I could feel his anxious, fidgety energy calming down. His face and his respiration relaxed. I kept singing and tapping until I sensed that he was in a state of deep relaxation.

After I finished, I had him lie on the sofa. He was silent, peaceful, and still for about a quarter of an hour. Then he started snoring. A few minutes later he sat up as if nothing had happened.

"Did you have a good nap?" I asked.

"I wasn't sleeping," he said.

"Well, you were certainly snoring," I told him.

"But I was seeing so much light, and vivid colors," he said, seeming puzzled, and thoughtful.

Dave said nothing else about his experience. I let him savor it. As he was leaving, he paused by the door. "I've been thinking about business way too much these days," he said. "It's like I forgot why I started this company. I did it because I believed in the healing power of herbs and I wanted to make them available to other people. But I've become obsessed with money and marketing."

Out of the mouth of the patient comes the perfect diagnosis, I thought.

"Why don't you have weekly meetings where you and your staff consider these kinds of things," I suggested, expanding on his own line of thinking. I knew by now how important it was to listen carefully to a patient, whose words often provide important clues to a remedy. Dave's words were clearly significant. "It's important to remember and share your belief in the value and purpose of your work," I said. "You could also brainstorm, or maybe share herbal healing stories. Staff meetings don't always have to be about sales numbers and bottom-line dollars."

I walked with him out to his car. On the way, I took a seedling from a patch of lemon balm in my front herb garden and gave it to him. Lemon balm is a subtle herb, mildly relaxing as a tea, with a soothing lemony smell. I wasn't sure how this meek little herb might help Dave's lion's roar of a problem. I told him to plant it in his garden and use it to make a tea for himself as often as he could. I was acting intuitively, as the "spirit" moved me. Who knows, perhaps I was guided by the spirit of the little herb itself. Dave took the plant, got into his rental car, and drove off to catch his plane.

Several months later, I received a phone call from Dave. He'd taken my suggestion on changing the focus of his staff meetings. As a result of this, he'd had two more customer-service lines installed in his office, and he'd instructed his staff to provide more in-depth, individualized support for their customers. These new staff meetings, and the more in-depth phone conversations between staff and clients, had strengthened the common bond of belief in the healing power of herbs between Dave and his staff and their customers. The result was a new level of customer loyalty. Sales had begun to climb. Also, Dave and his staff, now more centered in their ideals, and with a stronger sense of the value of their work, were happier on the job.

Not surprisingly, Dave also told me his stomach ulcers had disappeared without the aid of medications. He'd given his wife the little lemon balm seedling I'd given him, and she'd planted it in their garden. And occasionally, after returning home from a long day's work, they enjoyed a pot of fresh lemon balm tea.

It was clear to me that the most significant factor in Dave's healing was a shift in his perspective that resulted in a healthy change of lifestyle, one that brought him into harmony with his deeply held values and his sense of purpose. Dave's shift allowed him to achieve integrity in his business and personal life. That's what I'd call powerful "medicine" right there.

The spiritual Rx for Josie's depression was not Prozac but re-connecting with the healing power of nature. Prescription antidepressants and other conventional medications are useful in their proper place, but they are no substitute for the necessary spiritual component of the healing process.

Just so, anti-inflammatory medications were not the answer to my carpal tunnel condition. The deeper medicine I needed was making necessary life-changes, finding work I believed in, and recovering a sense of meaning and purpose in my life. In the same way, the spiritual Rx for my cancer was not surgery but finding my "voice" and learning to speak my truth. I am now both physically cancer-free and spiritually fear-free, free to tell my story just as I am doing now.

But how these healing shifts occur is part of the mystery of spirited medicine. It's often difficult to distinguish between primary and secondary healing factors. Where was the "medicine" in Dave and Josie's cases? Not in any pills, nor even merely in the herbs. Was Josie's depression healed primarily by the lavender, its oils, its smell, its spirit? Or was the primary healing factor working in a garden that connected her more directly to the forces (and spirits) of nature? There's no way to gauge precisely. The doctor hopes to find neat, concise explanations, so that specific healing procedures can be reliably repeated by others. The shaman embraces mystery, and performs specific healing procedures, trusting the medicine, and the power of spirit which he or she invokes.

So where does pharmaceutical/technological medicine end, and the work of spirited healing begin? As a pharmacist and a shamana—or a spirited healer—I walk in both worlds, seeking wholeness and healing every day. And I'm still learning, growing, practicing, asking questions, and seeking answers.

Spirited medicine is not a hard science, like chemistry, yet neither is it mystical voodoo. Spirited healers do not see man as the passive pawn of spirits who cause and cure his diseases. A spirited healer helps others to understand the psycho-physical roots of much illness, and helps them reconnect to the spiritual dimension and to the life-force that heals. In making diagnoses and prescribing remedies, a spirited healer considers the multi-dimensional nature of the patient—a being made of mind, body and spirit—then endorses both appropriate natural remedies, and the wise and necessary uses of medical science and technology.

The hubris of conventional medicine has been that it essentially views the body in mechanical terms, and so denies, in theory and in practice, the spiritual dimensions and needs of their patients, and the necessary spiritual components of both disease and the healing process. In its rigid denial of this spiritual dimension, it needlessly ties one hand behind its back. Such hubris is an old story.

The "germ theory" of disease was at first violently rejected by doctors, called superstition and quackery—at a time when bloodletting was still common practice, and surgeons didn't bother washing their hands before operating on their patients. No need to wash, since they *knew* germs didn't exist. Invisible, microscopic, disease-bearing critters crawling everywhere around us and inside us? Nonsense, the experts asserted with scorn. How many lives were harmed or lost before this important truth was finally accepted?

As we know, the "germ-theory" turned out to be one of mankind's most significant discoveries. Now I propose we consider a "spirit theory," too—a theory that allows for spiritual causes of illness. The kind of healing necessary in such cases is *spirited medicine by spirited healers.* The spiritual Rx given out would be a good dose of the same *invisible medicine* don Antonio had given me, but given out by our own Western healthcare practitioners and healers.

I believe we are now indeed in the process of recognizing, and implementing these important truths as contained in the spirited healing paradigm I've addressed in this book. There are a growing number of individuals, including healthcare practitioners, who ascribe to the principles of spirited healing. Once our medical institutions can "officially" recognize patients, and physicians, as spiritual/ emotional beings, they will also begin to recognize the tremendous healing power of a doctor's compassionate care and concern for each and every patient's physical and *spiritual* welfare. They will recognize the spiritual bond between patient and doctor as a vital part of the healing process. (Every child knows that a mother's hug removes the sting from a scraped knee.) And they will understand that the chemical management of symptoms, currently a widespread medical practice, is not the same as healing. When this shift comes about, conventional Western medicine will have grown from knowledge, to wisdom.

In the end, neither shaman nor scientist can fully explain the "magic" of healing, which resides in the realms of nature and spirit. What matters is that people are helped, healed, and spiritually enriched on the path they walk in life. Our own wholeness is the healing we all truly seek. All healing is ultimately mysterious. And maybe we all need a little more mystery in our lives.

EPILOGUE

I am now emerging from nearly a decade's apprenticeship to the spirits of the Amazon jungle, one of them being the rainforest shaman don Antonio. Pleased with my progress, and having recently released me from the rigorous dietas and disciplinas of my early apprenticeship, don Antonio says he has found in me—an ordinary middle-aged Western woman, and his only non-indigenous apprentice—someone to carry on his lineage of healing knowledge. He refers to me as "the blue-eyed, white shamana who has become the spirit of the jungle."

Who would have thunk?

I went to the Amazon in search of my own healing, and I became a shaman's apprentice to find the magic that was missing in my own healing tradition. There I was cooked in a cauldron of shamanic medicine rituals, disciplinas and un-usual life-experiences, and blown apart by the magnitude and mystery of spirit. In the end, this intense apprenticeship forced me to "let go." At some point, it became clearly more useful to open my mind, disregard my prejudices, and discover what works rather than continue stubbornly to cling to the superiority of my beliefs and presumptions. Letting go into the mystery has been a most liberating and humbling experience.

Now, as far from perfect and as ordinary as ever, I have no magic potions, no supernatural powers, and no ultimate answers. The only thing in my "bag of tricks" is me, and the healing knowledge I've been given by spirit and the mystery of life.

So, am I crazy like my mother after all? If I am, so be it. I have no regrets. In fact, I'm grateful. Because my life is deeper and more fulfilling than I ever imagined it could be. My mind and senses have been opened, at times painfully, to the spirit of things, to dimensions of life outside the box of conventional, consensus reality. Healing spirits appear to me and do their work. Plants talk to me, and give me useful information. The kinds of experiences that led my mother to her ruin, have expanded my horizons, enriched my life, and led me to greater wholeness. I sometimes think, sadly, that if she had only fallen into kinder, gentler, wiser hands than she did, what a shamana she might have made! But she had her own journey to take.

In my own journey, I had to fly halfway around the world, venture into the heart of the jungle, and become a sorcerer's apprentice to find the path, the wisdom, the experiences, that led me back to my own center where I could be healed. And what magical healing truths did I find? I found that the Earth, the plants, and the power of nature can heal us. I found that plants are living spirits with gifts to offer us. I found that life itself is the journey, the food and the medicine. All the medicine we need is right here beneath our feet. And in the end, all the paths we choose and the medicines we take are meant to return us to our center where the healing power of spirit dwells.

So when your life is a tough pill to swallow, remember, it's your medicine. My dull, repetitious, suffocating life of quiet desperation led me into the dark corridors of illness and despair, and out the other end into a new, passion-filled life. This is what spirit can do for us if we pay attention and follow its call. And when we dare to step outside the rigid patterns of our mechanistic lives to take new paths and follow new visions, we find our truer selves. We find a purpose that gives sparkle and verve to our lives, that fills us with the energy and spirit of life. If it happened to me, it can happen to you. A little plant, and spirit told me so. And a shaman named don Antonio.

So if you want the deepest healing and the greatest adventure, hop into your own spirit-guided canoe and journey along the mighty Amazon of life until you find the Garden of Eden that will feed your soul. And join me there in sipping a dose of spirited medicine from the cup of life itself.

Salud.

GLOSSARY

achiote – the tree *Bixa orellana* whose fruit is used by the indigenous as a red dye for body paint. At one time was FDA approved as Red Dye Number 3 food coloring, often used to tint cheese, butter, and rice. Various parts of the tree and its fruit are used to treat a wide range of illnesses.

abrazos – hugs.

agouti – a rabbit-sized rodent, related to the guinea pig.

aguardiente – local sugar cane rum, literally means "fire or burning water."

ajo sacha – wild garlic, *Mansoa alliacea*, used as medicine for arthritis and asthma, as well as for spiritual protection against evil spirits.

alumna – student.

arnica – a local common name for a plant that is known scientifically as *Cosmos* which we use as an ornamental, while the indigenous use it for a variety of medical conditions.

artesanía – contemporary native crafts of the Yagua.

Astrocaryum – *Astrocaryum chambira* or fiber palm, genus of palm trees which contains the species known locally as *chambira*.

au contraire – French for "to the contrary."

ayahuasca – in Quechua, means "vine of the dead" or "vine of the soul." Ayahuasca is both the name of the vine *Banisteriopsis caapi* itself, as well as the name of the multi-ingredient hallucinogenic brew commonly used by Amazonian shamans as medicine for divination and healing.

ayahuasquero – one who uses the ayahuasca liquid medicine to heal.

bien – fine.

calabash – bowl, made from the large fruits of the calabash tree, used as a bowl or a dipper, as well as decorative handicraft carvings.

camote – *Ipomoea batatas*, whose tubers are the edible sweet potato, while its leaf and other plant parts are used for a variety of medical conditions.

camu camu – *Myrciaria dubia*, edible fruit contains 10-20 times more vitamin C than any other known fruit; has the potential as a good crop for export as source for vitamin C.

capinurí – *Maquira coriacea*, large buttressed tree used in the production of plywood, as well as indigenous medicine to increase virility. Its phallic shaped branches are a good example of the Doctrine of Signatures.

casho – cashew, *Anacardium occidentale*, a tree whose nuts are edible, fruit juice is high in vitamin C; and whose other tree parts have a variety of medicinal and industrial uses.

cecropia – large rainforest tree, used to make medicine, as well as wood to make canoes and blowguns.

ceiba – giant kapok tree, *Ceiba pentandra*, highly prized for its wood and kapok. Overexploited to extinction in certain areas.

cena – dinner.

chambira – local name for a palm tree of the *Astrocaryum* genus of palms, prized for its fiber to make hammocks handbags, and ropes.

chonta – heart palm, *Euterpe precatoria*, prized for its delicious heart of palm. Beetles eggs laid in this tree become edible nutritious larvae grub worms called "suri", that are prized and eaten live by the natives.

clavo huasca – tasty clove vine, *Tynnanthus panurensis*, when mixed with *aguardiente* is used to energize a person as well as to treat rheumatism.

Cocama – indigenous tribe of Amazonia, don Antonio's native tribe.

cocamera – large round thatch-enclosed communal hut of the Yagua Indians.

colectivo – public river taxi.

copal – a yellowish tree resin from the *Copaifera reticulata* tree that is used medicinally to treat a variety of ailments, as well as an incense to purify a ritual area for ceremony.

cuidado – be careful!

curare – *Chondrodentron tomentosum*, when mixed with poison frogs and stinging ants, makes a toxic concoction used in hunting. Natives store it in tubes. This is the source of the pharmaceutical tubocurarine (hence the name) used in modern medicine. *Strychnos guianensis*, is an eastern Amazonian curare plant which has strychnine as its toxic component; and the indigenous store this kind of curare in pots.

curarina – *Potalia amara*, a plant whose mottled coloring on its trunk has given it the name of "snakebite plant", for which it is used medicinally. Classic example of Doctrine of Signatures.

cushma – a black shroud-like poncho, worn by the shaman in rituals.

datura – toé, *Brugmansia aurea* plant with large distinctive bell shaped flowers, hence the name "angel's trumpet." Its scopolamine-containing leaves are used as an additive of the arrow-poison curare, as well as an hallucinogenic additive to ayahuasca brew.

dieta – dietary restrictions followed by a shaman as part of their spiritual practice.

disciplina – lifestyle restrictions followed in a shaman's spiritual practice.

don – a term of respect, used in front of a male person's name; the feminine form would be doña.

energia positiva – positive energy or vital force, spirit.

finito – finished, you're dead!

gringo/gringa – North American man/woman.

guayusa – *Ilex guayusa*, the leaves of this plant are rich in caffeine. The Achuar Indians of Amazonia drink it every morning, to induce vomiting, as part of a daily cleansing ritual.

hierba luisa – lemon grass, *Cymbopogon citratus*, is an aromatic plant used as a relaxant as well as to treat headache, fever, and digestive problems.

huito – *Genipa americana*, blue-black dye squeezed from the fruits of the huito tree that is used as body paint, "jungle tattoos." It is also used medicinally for a variety of conditions by the indigenous.

ícaro – magical healing song that a shaman sings to his patients.

Inga – *Inga edulis*, or ice cream bean tree contains long bean pods, inside of which contains seeds coated with succulent sweet meat. The tree is said to have a variety of other medicinal properties as well.

Jacaranda – *Jacaranda* spp., tree whose wood is used for construction and pulp for paper; its leaves and other tree parts are used medicinally to treat numerous conditions.

limón – *Citrus aurantifolia*, a member of the lemon family used as medicine, as well as refreshing drink or food garnish.

limpia – ritual healing herbal bath, from the Spanish word "limpiar" which means "to clean."

Los Tres Mosqueteros – The Three Musketeers.

maestro – teacher.

magia – magic.

maloca – open round communal house.

mañana – tomorrow.

mapacho – black tobacco that is smoked during ayahuasca healings and cleansing rituals.

medicina – medicine.

mesa – table, in this context a shaman's holy altar adorned with sacred objects.

moriche – *Mauritia flexuosa*, a tree whose palm leaves are used to make fibers and roof thatch. Its fruits, *aguajes*, are eaten raw or as a fruit drink.

morpho – large iridescent blue quintessential butterfly of the tropics.

murcura – *Petiveria alliacea*, ritually used in a healing herbal bath is said to give *energia positiva*. Medicinally, it is used by the indigenous for a variety of ailments, such as rheumatism, worms, stings and bites.

no es broma – is no joke!

no hay problema – no problem!

Oropendola – golden tailed bird, whose nests resemble large pendulous drops.

paciencia – patience.

paiche – large Amazon river fish, reaching 10 feet and 200 pounds, prized as food.

paico – *Chenopodium ambrosioides*, an aromatic plant used medicinally to treat many conditions including fever, flu, stomachache, and worms.

papaya – a tree whose tasty fruit is rich in Vitamin C. The fruit is also used medicinally for its enzymes; its other tree parts are used medicinally to treat wounds and infections, amongst other uses.

pauraque – bird, member of the nightjar family with a distinctive wolf whistle call.

piñón blanco – *Jatropha curcas*, a shrub whose leaves are used to treat infections; and whose other plant parts are used medicinally for a variety of other conditions.

piranha – fish, famous and feared for its razor sharp teeth. Most species of piranha are omnivorous, some are vegetarians, and some are carnivores.

Plaza de Armas – Military Square in the center of the town of Iquitos.

plátano – plantain, larger banana, with a higher starch content suitable for frying or boiling. Plantains and bananas both contain high amounts of carbohydrates, vitamins, and calories; both a good source of nutrition in the tropics.

problema – problem.

pucuna – blowgun, named after the *Pucuna caspi* tree from which its made.

purga – purgative, that which causes vomiting and diarrhea.

qué es esta – what is this?

quinine – *Cinchona officinalis*, effective modern pharmaceutical treatment for malaria. Also used medicinally by the indigenous of South America.

rapido – high-powered speed boat.

resfriado – head cold.

ribereños – mestizos (mixed blood) living along the rivers of northeast Peru.

Rio Amazonas – Amazon River, named after the legendary fearsome women warriors of Greek mythology, purportedly because of the indigenous men in grass/fiber skirts that early explorers came across in this region.

salud – a toast which means "to your health."

sangre de grado – "dragon's blood", red sap of the *Croton lechleri* tree used medicinally both topically as a wound-healer as well as orally to treat bacterial diarrhea. Pharmaceuticals derived from this plant are currently in clinical trials.

selva – jungle, forest.

serpiente – snake, *el serpiente* means anaconda here.

sexo – sex.

shacapa – bouquet of plant leaves, used like a maraca, that flop and rattle (the name *shacapa* comes from the rhythmic sound of these leaves when beaten together) to keep rhythm during the shaman's singing of the *ícaros*.

tabaco – tobacco.

tambo – raised-platform, thatch-roofed shelters.

tamarin – small monkeys, eight to ten inches high weighing less than one pound.

tangarana – ant tree, a tree that houses ants which in turn protect the tree.

tigre – tiger, used here *el tigre* means "jaguar."

Titi – arboreal monkeys; small, only up to three pounds and one and one half feet high.

turista – tourist.

uña de gato – *Uncaria* spp., named "cat's claw" vine because of the paired claw-like tendrils that grow under the leaves of this popular medicinal herb. Widely used as a medicine in the Amazon for a variety of conditions, cat's claw is gaining a good reputation as an anti-inflammatory and immunostimulant in the U.S.. Popular in the States as a botanical remedy, scientists are now studying its possible effects on cancer.

vámonos – let's go!

Victoria regia – Queen Victoria giant Amazonian water lily, used medicinally to treat inflammations and rheumatism. Stem, seeds, and roots are edible. Large white flowers open at night, attracting beetles to pollinate. In the early hours just before daylight, the flower closes around these beetles who are then trapped. The white flower turns to purple the next day, and reopens at darkness releasing the trapped beetles.

Yagua – an Amerindian indigenous tribe of the northwest Amazon.

yuca – *Manihot esculenta*, known also as cassava or manioc, is a root used as a dietary source of starch/carbohydrate. Besides food, this root is also used to make an alcoholic beverage known as *masato*. Its roots contain a high concentration of cyanide, which is removed upon heating and cooking.

zapatos – shoes.

DRUGS
DERIVED NATURALLY
FROM PLANTS

Tropical plants in bold
*Drugs or herbs currently used in the U.S.

DRUG	SPECIES	ACTION/CLINICAL USE
Aesculetin	*Fraxinus rhynchophylla*	Dysentery
Andrographolide	***Andrographis paniculata***	**Dysentery**
Arecoline	***Areca catechu***	**Anthelmintic**
Asiaticoside	***Centella asiatica***	**Vulnerary**
Atropine*/ Hyoscyamine*	*Atropa belladonna*	**Anticholinergic**
Berberine*	*Berberis vulgaris* (barberry)	Dysentery
Bergenin	***Ardisia japonica***	**Antitussive**
Bromelain*	***Ananas comosus***	**Proteolytic**
Camphor*	***Cinnamomum camphora***	**Rubefacient**
Castor oil*	***Ricinus communis***	**Cathartic**
Cissampeline	***Cissampelos pareira***	**Muscle relaxant**
Cocaine*	***Erythroxylum coca***	**Local anesthetic**
Codeine*	*Papaver somniferum*	Analgesic
Curcumin*	***Curcuma longa* (turmeric)**	**Choleretic**
Cynarin*	*Cynara scolymus* (artichoke)	Choleretic

Digoxin*/ Digitoxin* .... *Digitalis lantata/purpurea* .... Cardiotonic

Diosgenin* .... *Dioscorea species* .... **Female contraceptive**

Emetine*/ Ipecac* .... *Cephaelis ipecacuanha* .... **Emetic**

Glaucarubine .... *Simarouba glauca* .... **Amoebicide**

Glaziovine .... *Ocotea glaziovii* .... **Antidepressant**

Gossypol .... *Gossypium species* .... **Male contraceptive**

Kawain* .... *Piper methysticum* (kava) .... **Tranquilizer**

L-Dopa* .... *Mucuna deeringiana* .... **Antiparkinsonism**

Monocrotaline .... *Crotalaria sessiliflora* .... **Antitumor (topical)**

Morphine* .... *Papaver somniferum* .... Analgesics

Nicotine .... *Nicotiana tabacum* .... **Insecticide**

Ouabain* .... *Strophanthus gratus* .... **Cardiotonic**

Papain*/Chymopapain* .. *Carica papaya* .... **Proteolytic**

Papaverine* .... *Papaver somniferum* .... Muscle relaxant

Phyllodulcin .... *Hydrangea macrophylla* .... Sweetener

Physostigmine* (Eserine) . *Physostigma venenosum* .... **Anticholinesterase**

Picrotoxin .... *Anamirta cocculus* .... **Analeptic**

Pilocarpine* .... *Pilocarpus jaborandi* .... **Parasympathomimetic**

Quinidine* .... *Cinchona spp* .... **Antiarrhythmic**

Quinine* .... *Cinchona spp* .... **Antimalarial**

Quisqualic Acid .... *Quisqualis indica* .... **Anthelminthic**

Reserpine* .... *Rauwolfia serpentina* .... Antihypertensive

Rhomitoxin .... *Rhodondendron molle* .... Antihypertensive

Rorifone .... *Rorippa indica* .... **Antitussive**

Rotenone .... *Lonchocarpus nicou* .... **Piscicide**

Santonin .... *Artemisia maritima* .... Ascaricide

Scopolamine* .... *Datura metel* .... Sedative

Silymarin* .... *Silybum marianum* (milk thistle) .... Antihepatotoxic

SP303/ *Croton lechleri** .... *Croton lechleri* (sangre de grado) ... Antidiarrheal

Stevioside* .... *Stevia rebaudiana* (stevia) .... Sweetener

Strychnine .... *Strychnos nux-vomica* .... CNS stimulant

Theobromine* .... *Theobroma cacao* .... Diuretic

Trichosanthin .... *Trichosanthes kirilowii* .... Abortifacient

Tubocurarine* .... *Chondodendron tomentosum* ..... Muscle relaxant

Valepotriates* .... *Valeriana officinalis* (valerian) ...... Sedatives

Vasicine (Peganine) ..... *Adhatoda vasica* .... Oxytoxic

Vinblastine*/ Vincristine* . *Catharanthus roseus* .... Antineoplastic

Yohimbine* .... *Pausinystalia yohimba* .... Aphrodisiac

Yuanhuacine .... *Daphne genkwa* .... Abortifacient

Partial list, modified and updated data from:

DerMarderosian, Ara, Ph.D., and Gruber, John. 1996. *Back to the Future: Traditional Medicinals Revisited, Laboratory Medicine*, Vol. 27, No. 2: American Society of Clinical Pathologists.

Soejarto, D.D., Ph.D., and Farnsworth, N.R.. 1989. *Tropical Rainforests: Potential Sources for New Drugs?* Perspectives in Biology and Medicine.

R€F€R€N(€$
∆ND ∆DDITION∆L
R€$OUR(€$

Chapter 1: The Jungle Calls

A story in pictures of how pharmacy, botany, and medicine are historically inextricably bound together to make the foundation of our modern medicine.

- ○ Bender, G.A., and Thom, R.A. 1998. *A Pictorial History of Herbs in Medicine & Pharmacy.* Herbalgram No. 42. Austin, TX: American Botanical Council.

Chapter 2: Into the Garden of Eden

Ethnobotanists share their exciting adventures of jungle exploration and encounters with the shamans of Amazonia, as they look for plants as potential new pharmaceutical drug discoveries.

- ○ Plotkin, Mark, Ph.D.. 1994. *Tales of a Shaman's Apprentice.* New York, NY: Penguin Books.

- ○ Davis, Wade, Ph.D.. 1997. *One River: Explorations and Discoveries in the Amazon Rain Forest.* New York, NY: Simon & Schuster.

Experts document the indigenous uses of the medicinal plants of the Peruvian Amazon rainforest.

○ Duke, James Alan, Ph.D., and Vasquez, Rodolfo. 1994. *Amazonian Ethnobotanical Dictionary*. Boca Raton, FL: CRC Press.

○ Castner, J.L., Ph.D., Timme, S.L., and Duke, J.A... 1998. *A Field Guide to Medicinal and Useful Plants of the Upper Amazon*. Gainesville, FL: Feline Press.

○ Mejia, Kember, and Rengifo, Elsa. 2000. *Plantas Medicinales de Uso Popular en la Amazonía Peruana*. Lima, Peru: Tarea Asociación Gráfica Educativa.

Indigenous Amazonians of Peru keep alive their knowledge and use of medicinal plants in their gardens and surrounding forests.

○ Mustalish, Roger, Ph.D., and Baxter, Rebecca. 2001. *Mina Jao: A Village Green Pharmacy in Amazonia*. Herbalgram No. 51, Austin, TX: American Botanical Council.

○ McKeon, Kathy. 1995. *A Ribereños Garden*. Herbalgram. Austin, TX: American Botanical Council.

○ Hutchison, Jay. 1995. *On the Amazonian Trail of Useful Plants*. Herbalgram. Austin, TX: American Botanical Council.

The importance of ethnobotanical approaches to pharmaceutical drug discovery, as scientists continue the search into our rainforests for cures to treat our most difficult diseases.

○ Cox, P.A., Ph.D.. 2000. *Will Tribal Knowledge Survive the Millennium?* Vol. 287: Science.

○ Wagner, Daniel T., R.Ph.. 2000. *Tropical Remedies.* Nutrition Science News. New Hope Natural Media.

○ Phillipson, D.J.. 1997. *New Drugs from Old Plants.* Vol. 22, No. 2.: Herbs.

○ DerMarderosian, Ara, Ph.D., and Gruber, John. 1996. *Back to the Future: Traditional Medicinals Revisited,* Laboratory Medicine, Vol. 27, No. 2: American Society of Clinical Pathologists.

○ Tyler, Varro E., Ph.D..1995. *Plant Drugs, Healing Herbs & Phytomedicinals: Rainforest Conference Keynote Address.* Herbalgram. Austin, TX: American Botanical Council.

○ Cox, A., Ph.D., and Balick, Michael J.. 1994. *The Ethnobotanical Approach to Drug Discovery.* Scientific American.

○ Huxtable, Ryan, Ph.D.. 1992. *The Pharmacology of Extinction.* Vol. 37, No. 1: Journal of Ethnopharmacology.

○ Simon, John. 1992. *Tales from the Healing Forest.* Vol. 6, No. 3: UU World, Journal of the Unitarian Universalist Association.

○ Findeisen, Christina. 1991. *Natural Products Research and the Potential Role of the Pharmaceutical Industry in Tropical Forest Conservation*. Report prepared for the Periwinkle Project of the Rainforest Alliance.

○ Schultes, R.E., Ph.D.. 1991. *Dwindling Forest: Medicinal Plants of the Amazon*. Vol. 65, No. 1: Harvard Medical Alumni Bulletin.

○ Balick, Michael J., Ph.D.. 1990. *Ethnobotany and the Identification of Therapeutic Agents from the Rainforest*. Ciba Foundation symposium on the Bioactive Compounds from Plants.

○ Schultes, R.E., Ph.D.. 1990. *Gifts of the Amazon Flora to the World*. Vol. 50, No. 2: Arnoldia.

○ Soejarto, D.D., Ph.D., and Farnsworth, N.R.. 1989. *Tropical Rainforests: Potential Sources for New Drugs?* Perspectives in Biology and Medicine.

○ Plotkin, Mark, Ph.D.. 1988. *Conservation, Ethnobotany, and the Search for New Jungle Medicines: Pharmacognosy Comes of Age...Again*. Vol. 8, No. 5: Pharmacotherapy.

○ Weiss, Rudolph Fritz, M.D.. 1988. *Proof of the Efficacy of Plant Drugs*. Herbal Medicine, 6th Edition. Beaconsfield, England: Beaconsfield Publishers, Ltd.

○ Tyler, Varro E., Ph.D.. 1986. *Plant Drugs in the 21st Century*. Vol. 40, No. 3: Economic Botany.

○ Farnsworth, Norman R., Ph.D., Akerele, D., et al, 1985. *Medicinal Plants in Therapy*. Vol. 63, No. 6: Bulletin of the World Health Organization.

Superstitions and stories of the spirits of the Amazon, as recounted by locals.

○ Beaver, Milly, and Beaver, Paul. 1989. *Tales of the Peruvian Amazon*. Largo, FL: AE Publications.

Chapter 3: Losing my Mind...Coming to my Senses

A fascinating look at the healing properties of the spirits of plants, insights to the energetic lives of plants, as well as our human-plant connection.

○ Dossey, Larry, M.D.. 2001. *Being Green: On the Relationships Between People and Plants*. Vol. 7, No. 3: Alternative Therapies.

○ Cowan, Elliot. 1995. *Plant Spirit Medicine*. Newberg, OR: Swan Raven & Company.

○ Tompkins, Peter, and Bird, Christopher, 1989. *The Secret Life of Plants*. New York, NY: Harper and Row, Publishers.

Chapter 4: Death and Rebirth

Modern psychiatry and transpersonal psychology explore the importance of the journey of the spirit/psyche in the transformation of the Self.

○ Grof, Stanislav, M.D.. 1988. *The Adventure of Self-Discovery*. Albany, NY: State University of New York Press.

○ Metzner, Ralph. Ph.D.. 1998. *The Unfolding Self.*
Novato, CA: Origin Press.

○ Grof, Stanislav, M.D.. 1985. *Beyond the Brain.*
Albany, NY: SUNY Press.

The healthful benefits and therapeutic applications of
herbs and other natural medicines as alternative choices in
healthcare.

○ Weil, Andrew, M.D.. 1990. *Natural Health, Natural
Medicine.* Boston, MA: Houghton Mifflin.

○ Duke, James A., Ph.D.. 1997. *The Green Pharmacy.*
Emmaus, Pennsylvania: Rodale Press.

○ Weil, Andrew, M.D.. 1989. *A New Look at Botanical
Medicine.* No. 64: Whole Earth Review.

○ ANMP: Association of Natural Medicine Pharmacists:
www.anmp.org.

Chapter 5: Jungle Medicine

Healing stories of the medicinal uses of rainforest
plants and the shamans who use them.

○ Arvigo, Rosita. 1995. *Sastun.* San Francisco, CA:
Harper Collins.

○ Grauds, Constance. 1999. *Jungle Medicine...original
pharmacy.* Vol. 4, No. 4, The Source: Association of
Natural Medicine Pharmacists.

Chapter 6: Apprenticeship to the Vine of the Dead

A look at the medicine of divination and healing—
ayahuasca: chemistry, visionary paintings, anthropological

reports of uses by indigenous shamans, as well as personal stories of healing and transformation.

○ Metzner, Ralph, Ph.D.. 1999. *Ayahuasca: Hallucinogens, Consciousness, and the Spirit of Nature*. New York, NY: Thunder's Mouth Press.

○ Luna, Luis Eduardo, Ph.D., and Amaringo, Pablo. 1993. *Ayahuasca Visions: The Religious Iconography of a Peruvian Shaman*. Berkeley, CA: North Atlantic Books.

○ Lamb, Bruce F. 1974. *Wizard of the Upper Amazon: The Story of Manuel Cordova-Rios*. Berkeley, CA: North Atlantic Books.

○ Dobkin de Rios, Marlene, Ph.D.. 1972. *Visionary Vine*. Prospect Heights, IL: Waveland Press, Inc.

○ Lopez Vinatea, Luis A., Ph.D.. 2000. *Plants Used by Amazon Shamans in the Ayahuasca Drink*. Iquitos, Peru.

○ Luna, Luis Eduardo, Ph.D.. *Vegetalismo: Shamanism Among the Mestizo Population of the Peruvian Amazon*. Stockholm, Sweden: Almquist & Wiksell International.

Scientists report insights as to the nature of reality through the use of ayahuasca.

○ Narby, Jeremy, Ph.D.. 1998. *The Cosmic Serpent: DNA and the Origins of Knowledge*. New York, NY: Jeremy P. Tarcher.

○ Wolf, Fred Alan, Ph.D.. 1991. *The Eagle's Quest*, New York, NY: Touchstone.

A thorough investigation of shamanism and its many forms as practiced throughout the world.

○ Eliade, Mircea., Ph.D.. 1974. *Shamanism: Archaic Techniques of Ecstasy*. Princeton, NJ: Princeton University Press.

The origins of the hallucinogenic uses of plants found worldwide, as researched by our pioneers and leading experts.

○ Schultes, Richard Evans, Ph.D., and Hofmann, Albert. 1979. *Plants of the Gods: Origins of Hallucinogenic Use*. Maidenhead, England: McGraw-Hill Book Company.

Continuing scientific research on the benefits of ayahuasca and other psychedelics.

○ Callaway, J.C., Ph.D., D.J. McKenna, C.S. Grob, et al. 1999. *Pharmacokinetics of Ayahuasca alkaloids in Healthy Humans*. Vol. 65: Journal of Ethnopharmacology.

○ Nichols, David E., Ph.D., Editor. 1998. *The Heffter Review of Psychedelic Research*. Santa Fe, NM: The Heffter Research Institute.

○ MAPS: Multidisciplinary Association for Psychedelic Studies: www.maps.org.

Articles of interest on ayahuasca.

○ Plotkin, Mark J., Ph.D.. 2000. *In Search of Amazonian Plant Masters and the Healing Spirit of Ayahuasca*. Shaman's Drum. Williams, OR: Cross-Cultural Shamanism Network.

○ Metzner, Ralph, Ph.D.. 1999. *Ayahuasca and the Greening of Human Consciousness*. Shaman's Drum. Williams, OR: Cross-Cultural Shamanism Network.

Audio and video tapes from conference on ayahuasca.

○ Grauds, Constance, R.Ph.. 2000. *Apprenticeship in Amazonian Plant Spirit Healing*, professionally recorded presentations of Grauds and others at the Ayahuasca: Amazonian Shamanism, Science and Spirituality Conference. San Francisco, CA. www.conferencerecording.com.

Chapter 7: Spirit Doctors

A thorough accounting of the practices of Peruvian coastal shamanism and Andean mysticism, as told through personal transformational experiences of these women.

○ Jenkins, Elizabeth. 1998. *Initiation: A Woman's Spiritual Adventure in the Heart of the Andes*. New York, NY: Berkeley Publishing Group a member of Penguin Putnam Inc.

○ Glass-Coffin, Bonnie, Ph.D.. 1998. *The Gift of Life: Female Spirituality and Healing in Northern Peru*. University of New Mexico Press.

An American's story of dedication to spirit and his shamanic apprenticeship in the Huichol tradition.

○ Pinkson, Tom, Ph.D.. 1995. *Flowers of Wiricuta: A Gringo's Journey to Shamanic Power*. Mill Valley, CA: Wakan Press.

Chapter 8: The Shaman and The Surgeon

Western physicians discuss the importance of the mind/body factor in the healing equation.

- Dossey, Larry, M. D.. 1999. *Reinventing Medicine: Beyond Mind-Body to a New Era of Healing.* New York, NY: HarperCollins.

- Weil, Andrew, M.D.. 1995. *Spontaneous Healing.* New York, NY: Fawcett Columbine.

- Chopra, Deepak, M.D.. 1989. *Quantum Healing: Exploring the Frontiers of Mind/Body Medicine.* New York, NY: Bantam Books.

- Schulz, Mona Lisa, M.D.. 1998. *Awakening Intuition: Using Your Mind-Body Network for Insight and Healing.* New York, NY: Crown Publishing Group.

ABOUT THE AUTHOR AND HER WORK

Connie Grauds, R.Ph., stands with her feet firmly planted in two very different worlds.

For over thirty years she has worked as a pharmacist in the world of conventional western medicine. And, for nearly a decade Grauds has also worked as a shamana in the world of "non-rational" healing. In 1994 she apprenticed to an Amazonian shaman in the jungles of Peru where she learned the ancient healing art of spirited medicine.

Seeking to bring these two unique worlds closer to one another, Grauds founded the Center for Spirited Medicine (www.spiritedmedicine.com), dedicated to the globalization of sustainable medicines and the teaching of indigenous healing practices.

Her life work and passion focuses on integrating the healing aspects of plants into western medicine, and the spiriting of healthcare. She is President of the Association of Natural Medicine Pharmacists (www.anmp.org), and Assistant Professor of Clinical Pharmacy at the University of California, San Francisco. She also serves as Ajunct Faculty at the University of Minnesota, Center for Spirituality and Healing.

As a healer, Grauds teaches the spirited medicine of Amazonian shamanism world-wide. Call or write for information about workshops, retreats, speaking engagements, consulting and books.

The Center for Spirited Medicine
PO Box 150727
San Rafael, CA 94915
(415) 479-1512 ❖ www.spiritedmedicine.com

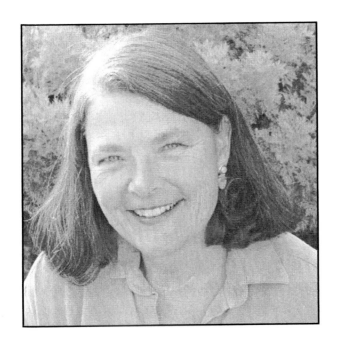

OTHER BOOKS BY CONNIE GRAUDS, R.PH.

*Energia Positiva...Nature's Prescription
for a Radiant, Healthy Life*

(Bantam Books, 2004)